SHAKY TOWN,

MY LIFE WITH PARKINSON'S DISEASE!

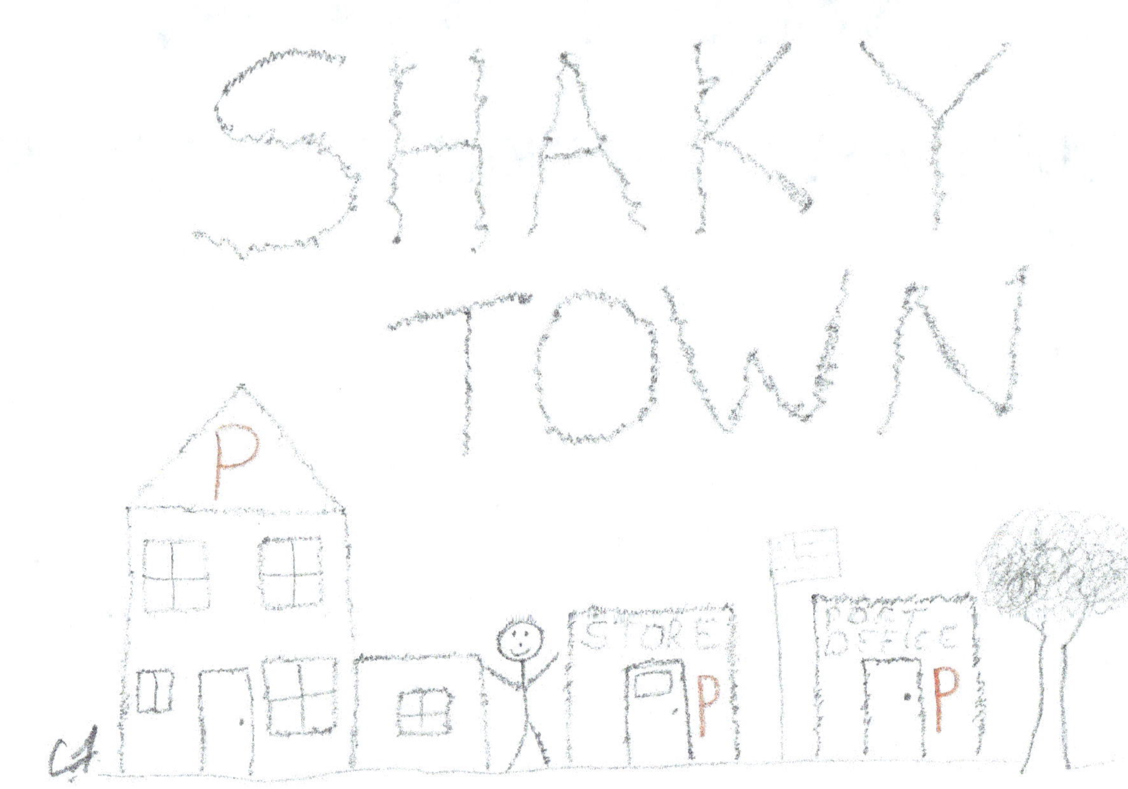

SHAKY
TOWN
P
STORE
POST OFFICE
P
P
P
P

Written and Illustrated

By Craig Fisher

I was diagnosed in 2020 with Parkinson's, and it really shocked the hell out of me.

I am not a Dr., and will not try to give any medical advice.

I am just expressing my feelings about the whole thing.

Parkinson's is different for
everybody, and everybody
handles it differently.
This is how I deal with it, and
Hopefully will help someone
down the line.

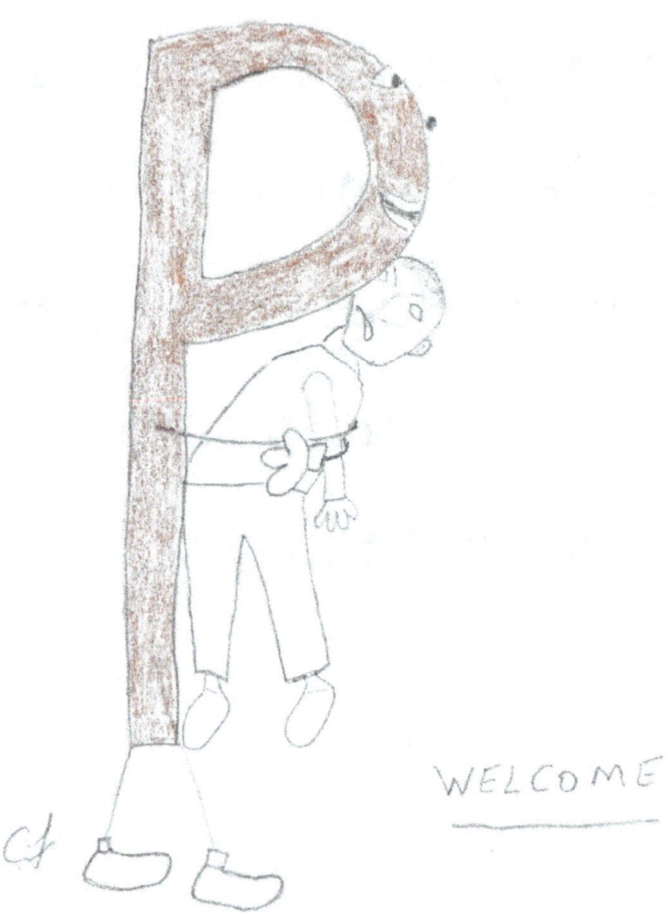
WELCOME

So, you have just been diagnosed with Parkinson's Disease, WELCOME!

I say that tongue in cheek because there is nothing welcoming about PD.

The Disease comes busting through and hits you like a ton of bricks!

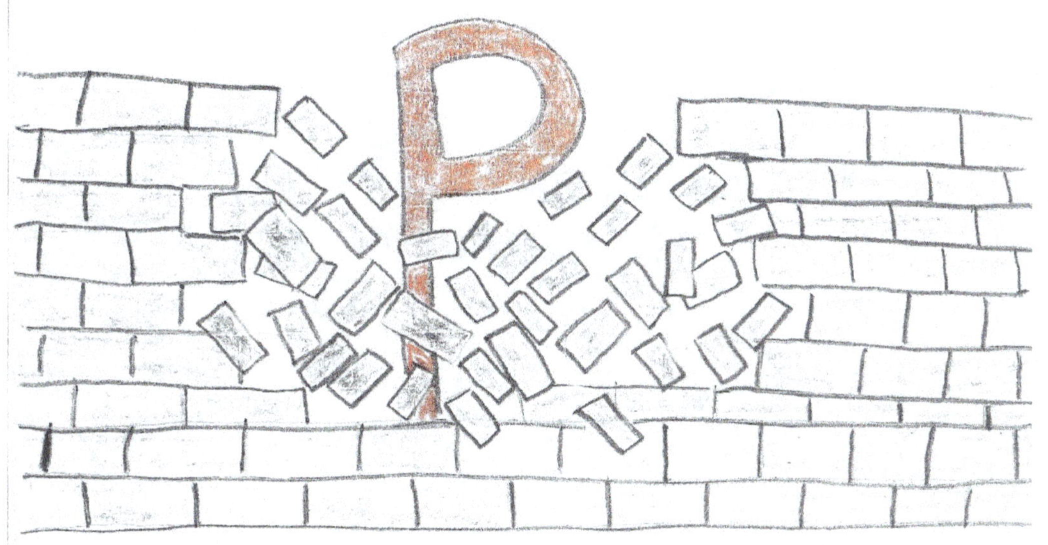

BUSTING THRU

Your life will now be a new type of life,

but one worth fighting for!

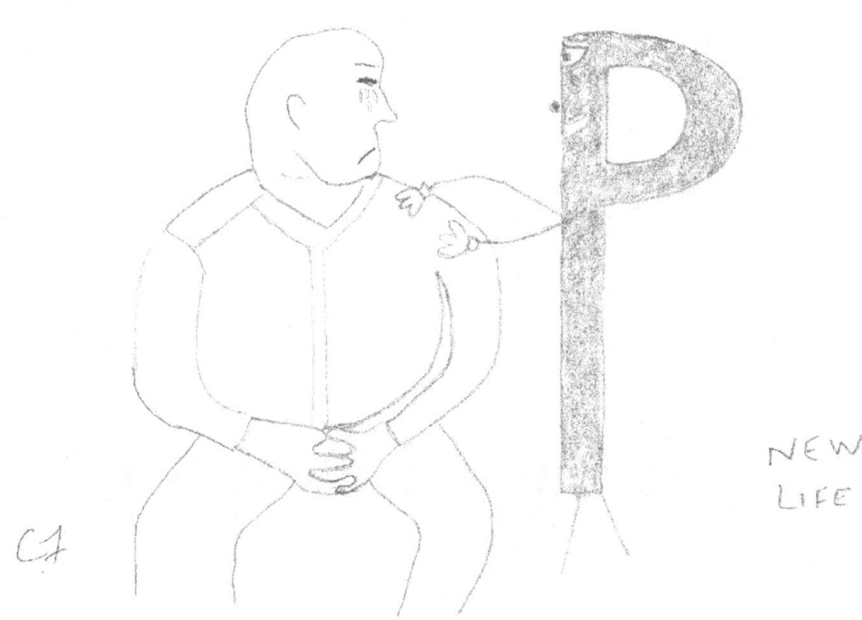

C1

You will wrestle with it,

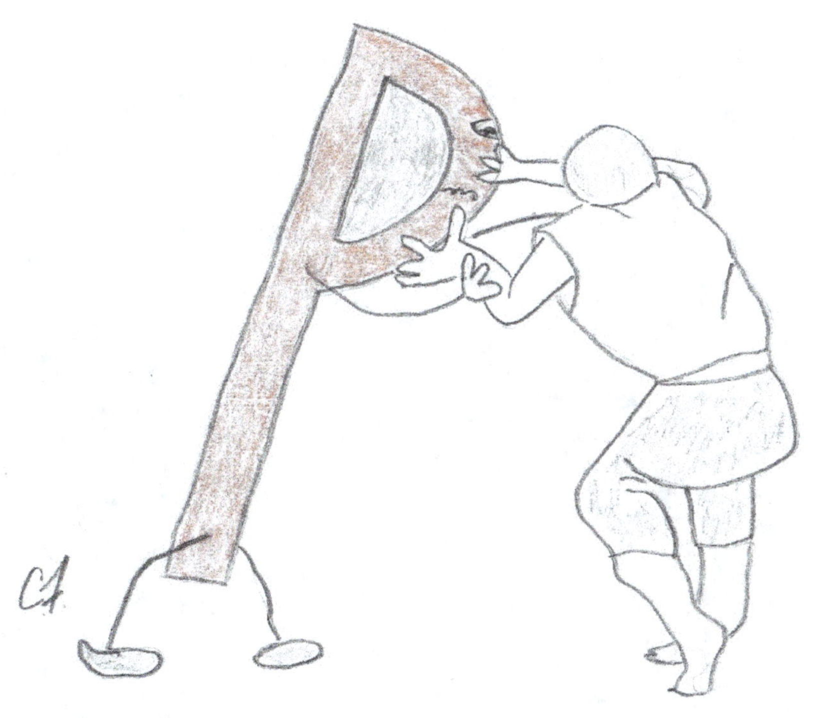

fight it,

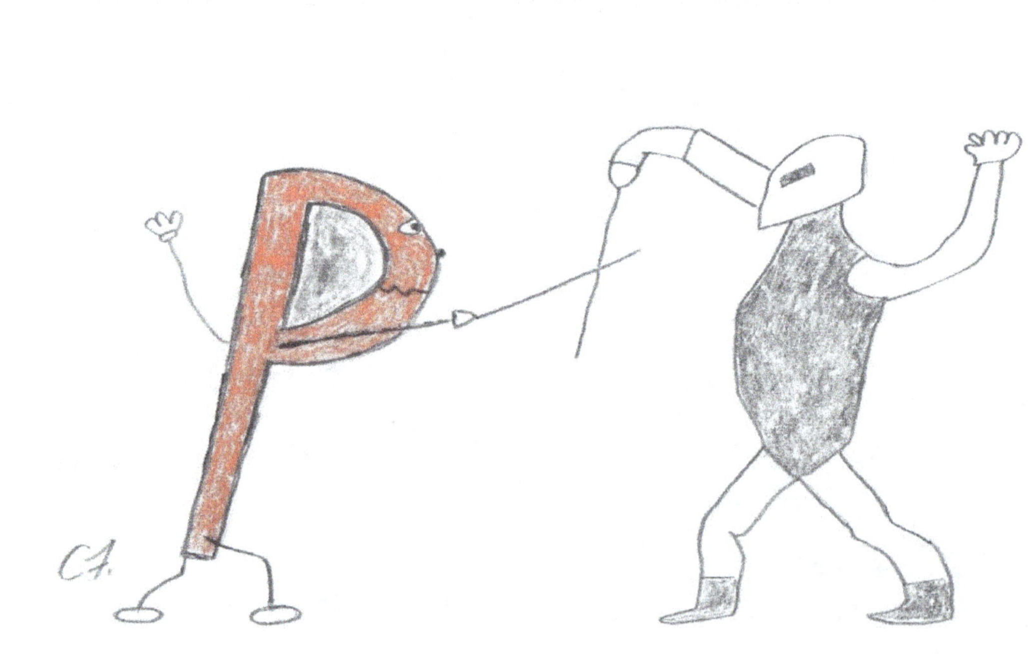

and even try to escape it, but to no avail.

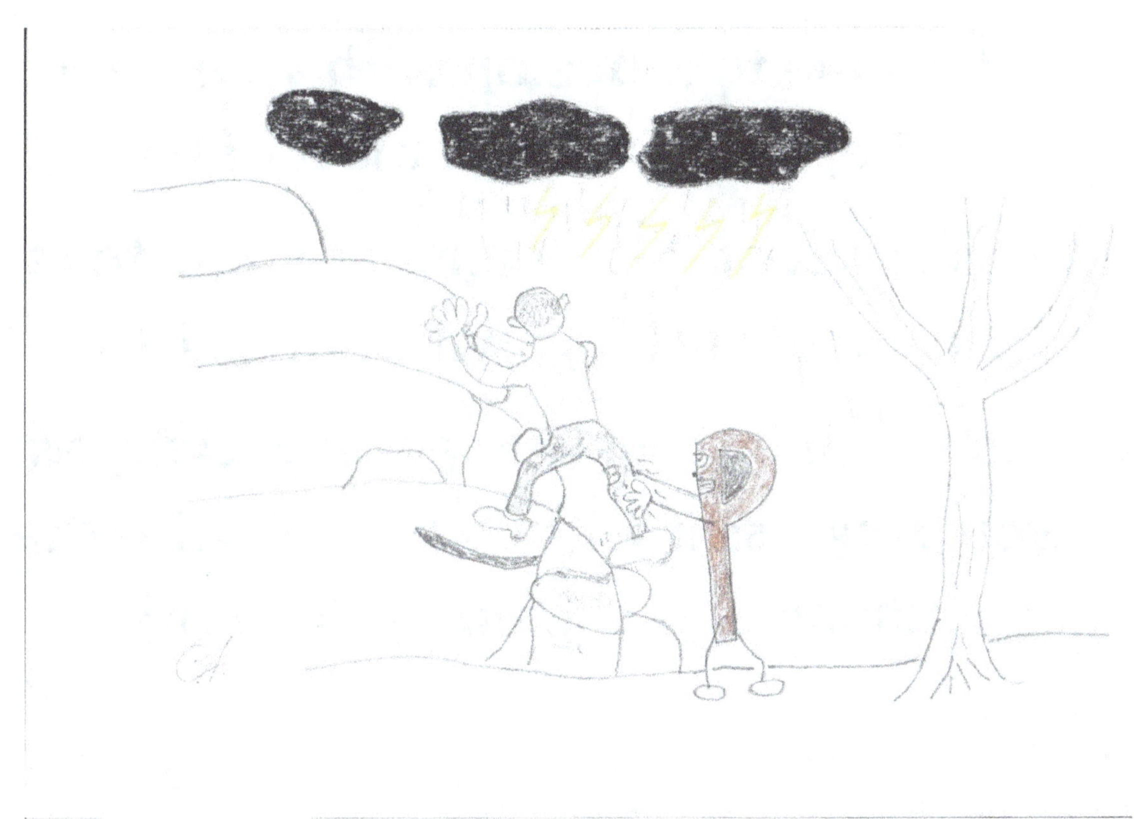

There is no escaping it!

It is time to move on with your new life, and make the most of it.

My mind set of it is; "I am not going to let it control my life, I will control it!"

Many things will change, especially as you progress it with, but work with the changes and keep having fun!

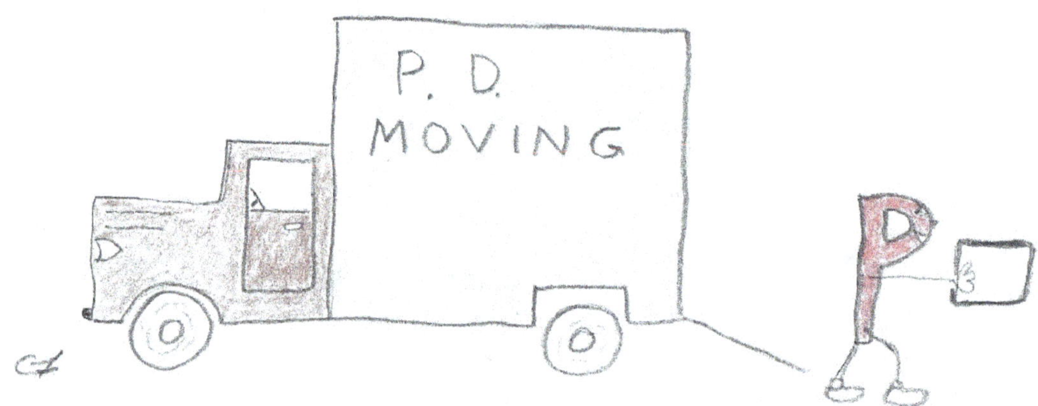

P. D.
MOVING

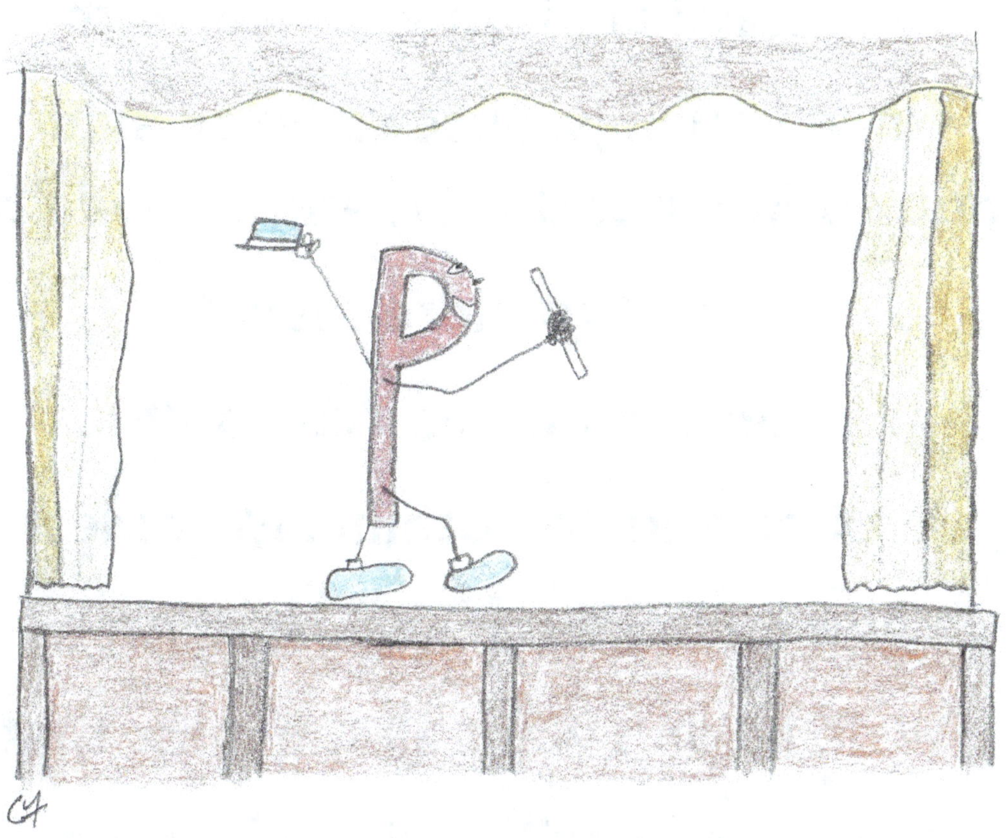

No, it is not all song and dance, but at the same time you cannot let it stop you!

We still want to live and have fun.
One way I am trying to deal with it is my drawings. I use to be an avid woodworker, but the Dr. and my wife both said "No more saws!"
I had to do something, I couldn't just sit around and do nothing. My oldest granddaughter suggested Art!
Well, I didn't want all the mess that comes along with paint, so thought I would try drawing.
It has helped tremendously!!!

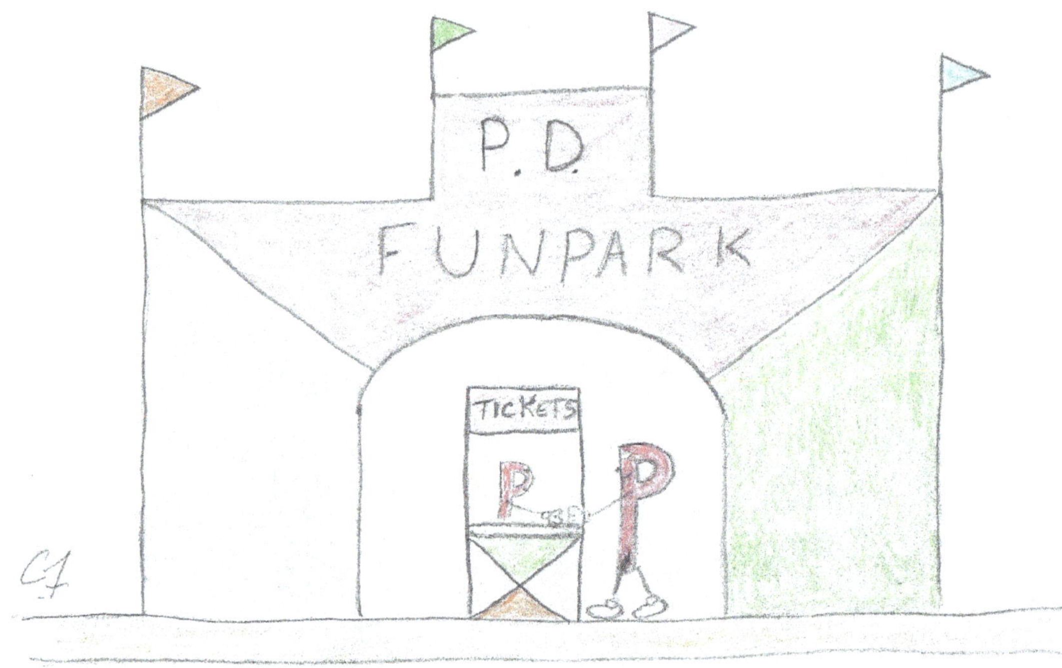

What can be more fun than going to a Fun Park?

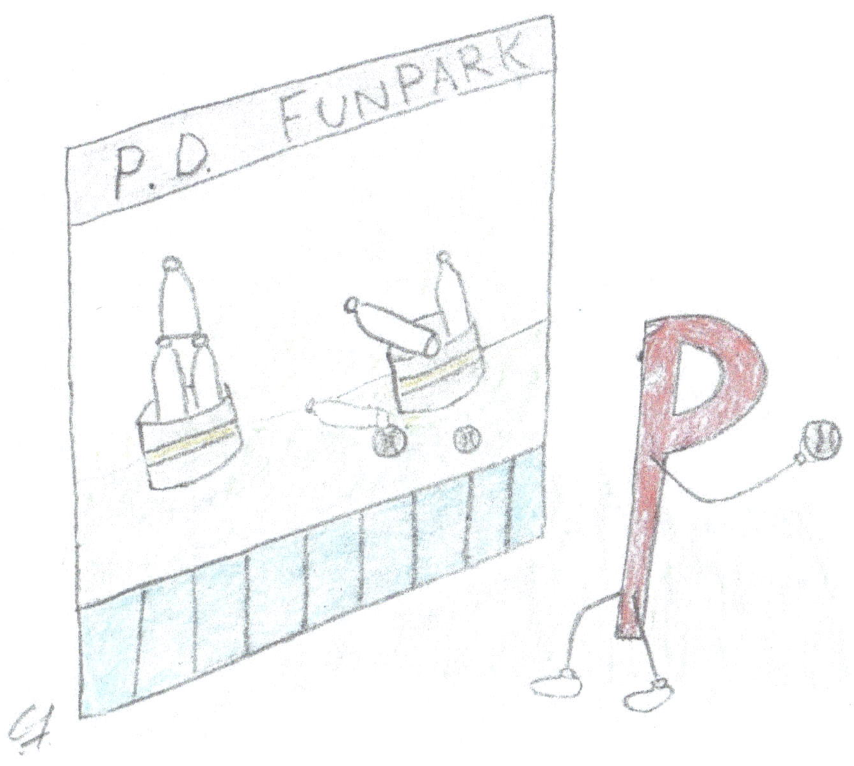

Play some games.

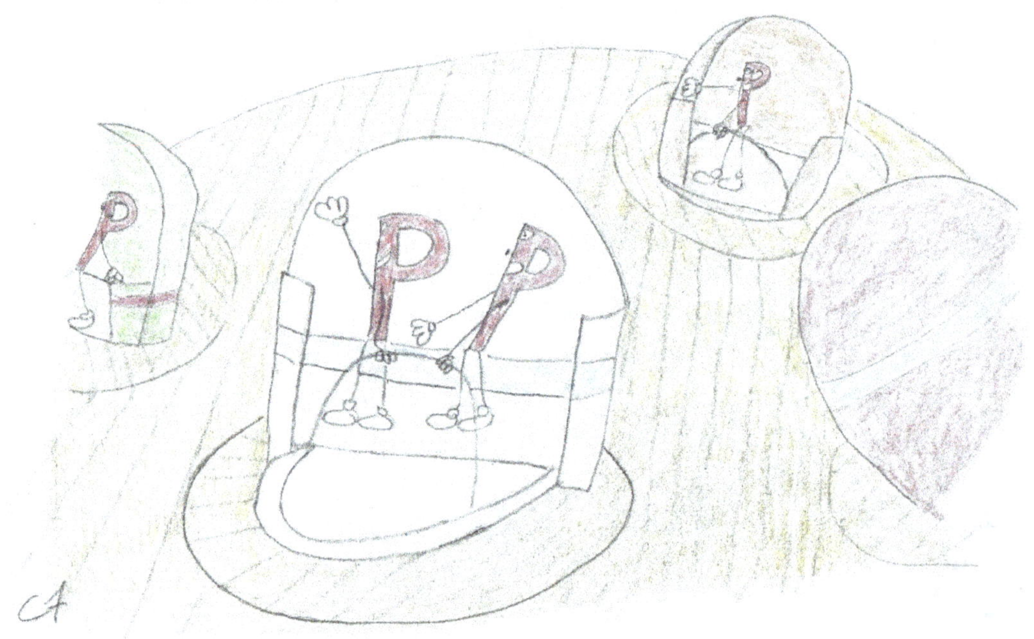
P.D. FUNPARK

Ride the rides.

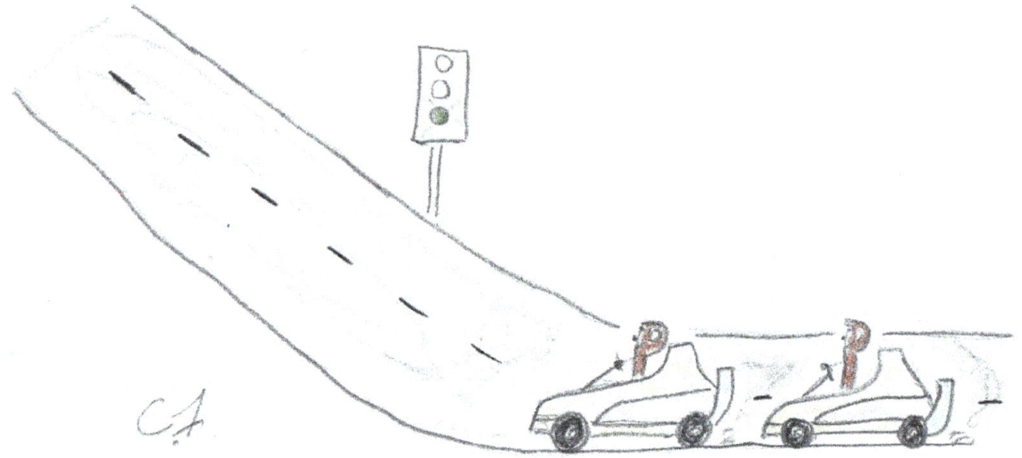

P.D. FUNPARK

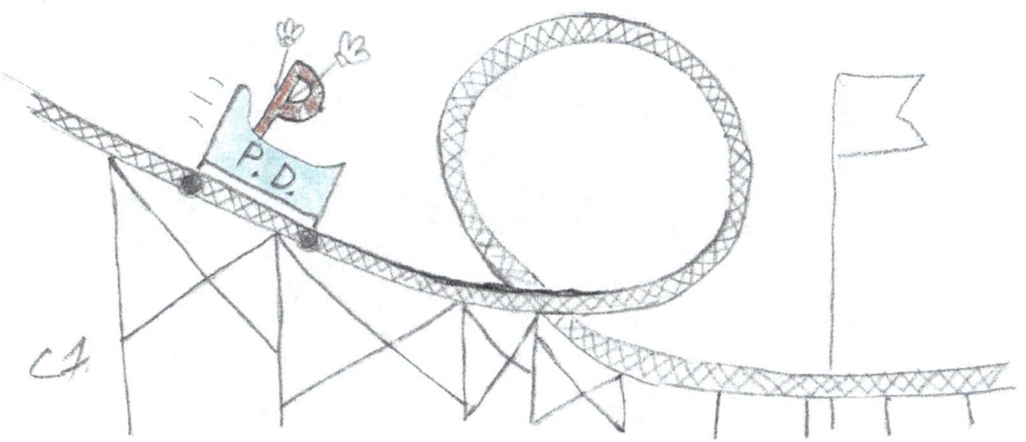

P.D. FUNPARK
P.D.

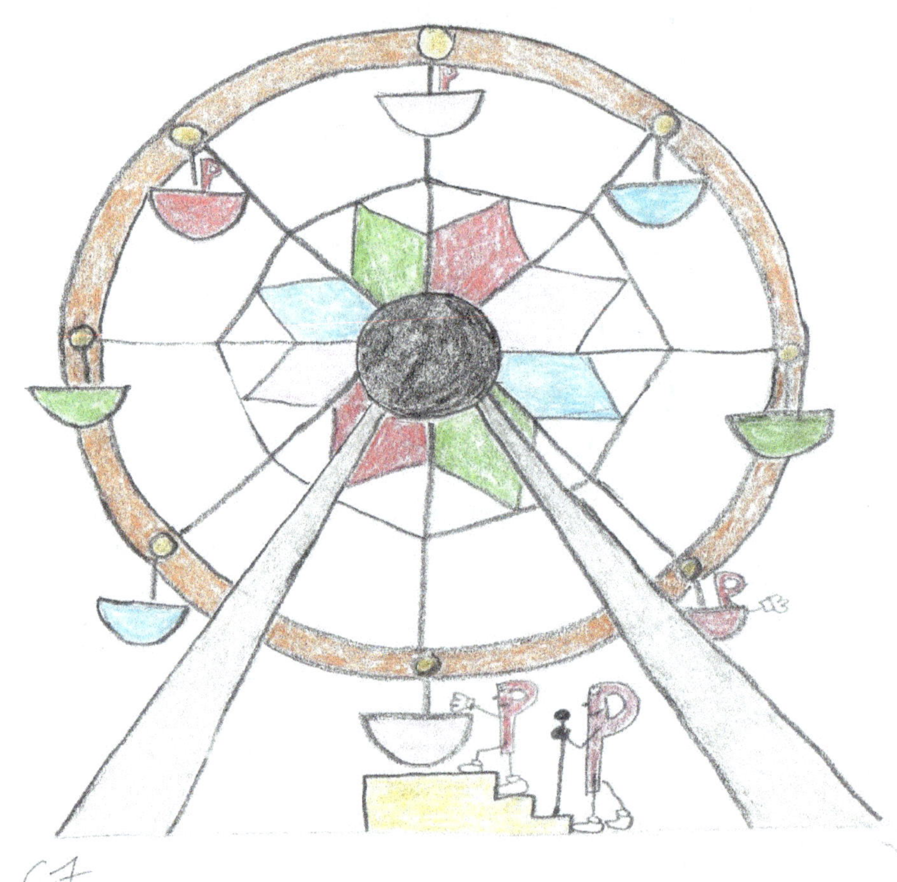

P.D. FUNPARK

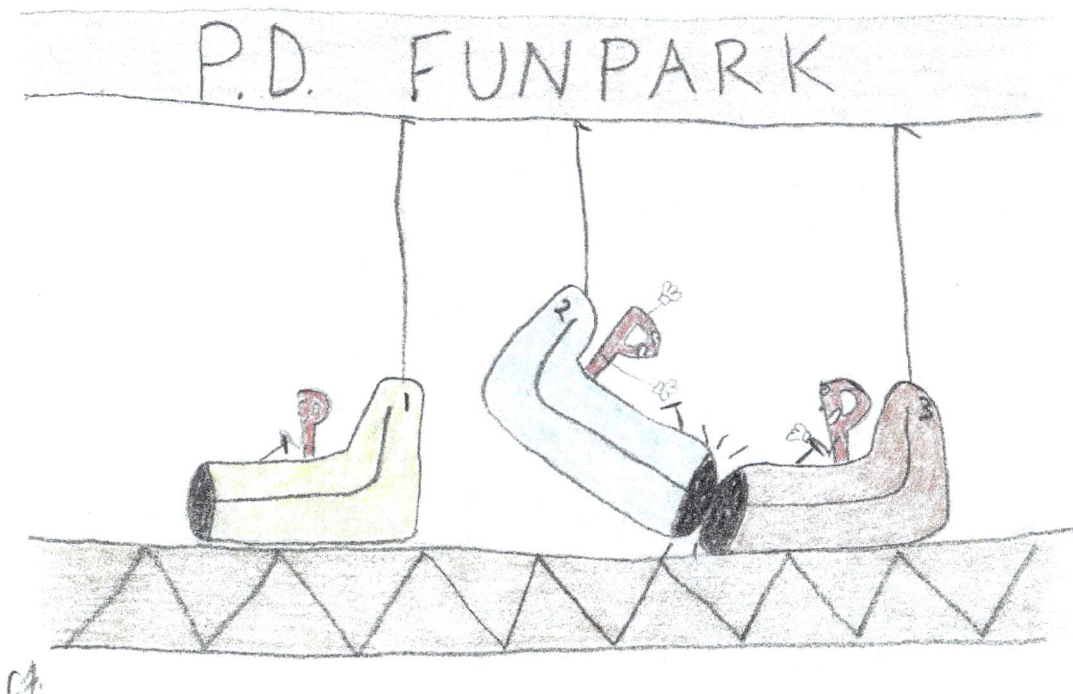
P.D. FUNPARK

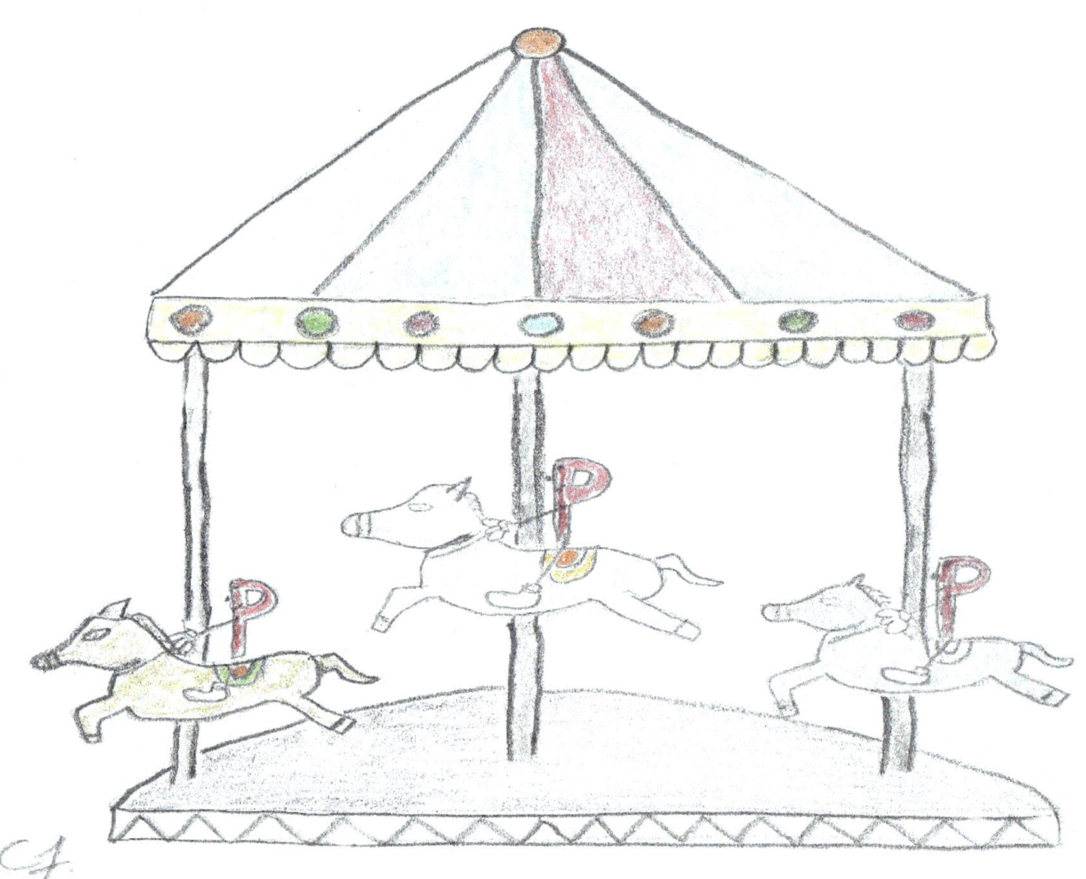
P. D. FUNPARK
P
P
P

P.D. FUNPARK

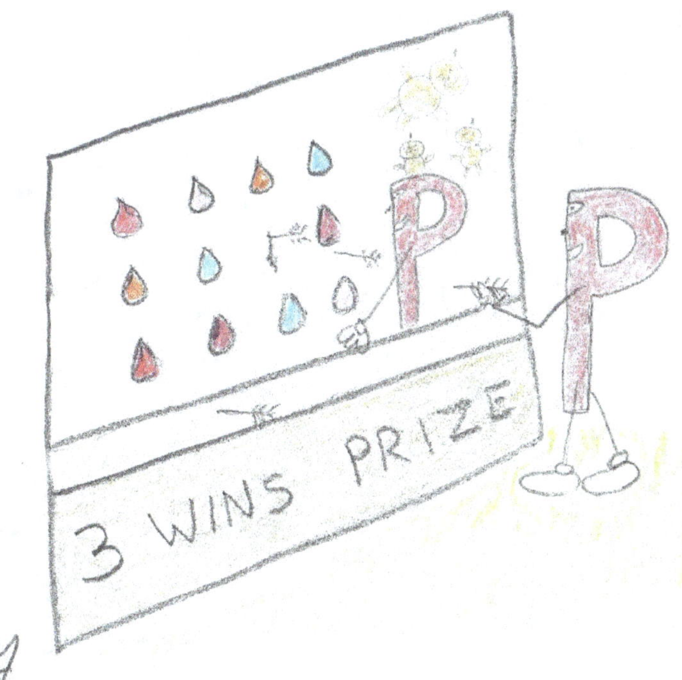

P
P
3 WINS PRIZE

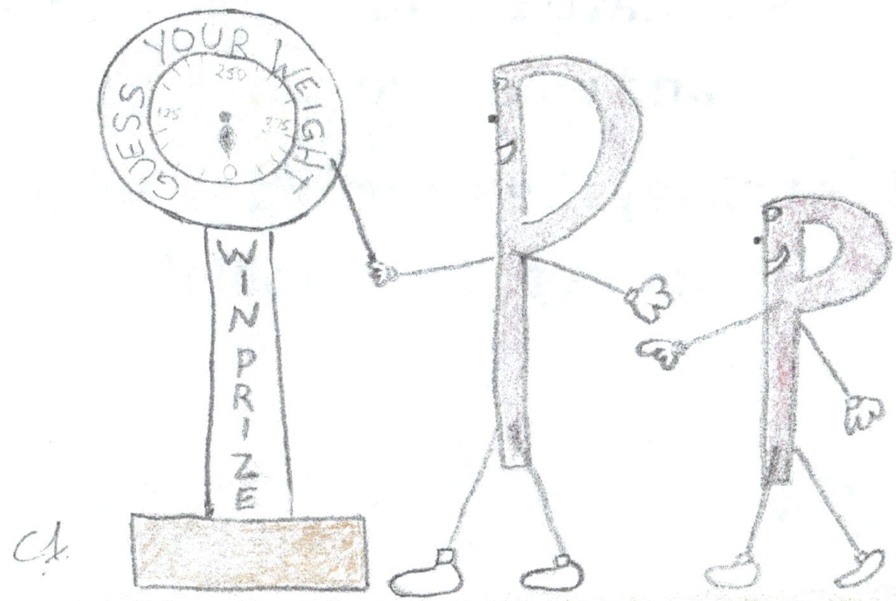

P.D. FUNPARK
GUESS YOUR WEIGHT
250
375
WIN PRIZE

We have to have our fun while we can,
and when we can.

It will not always be easy to deal with, but
we have to keep going!

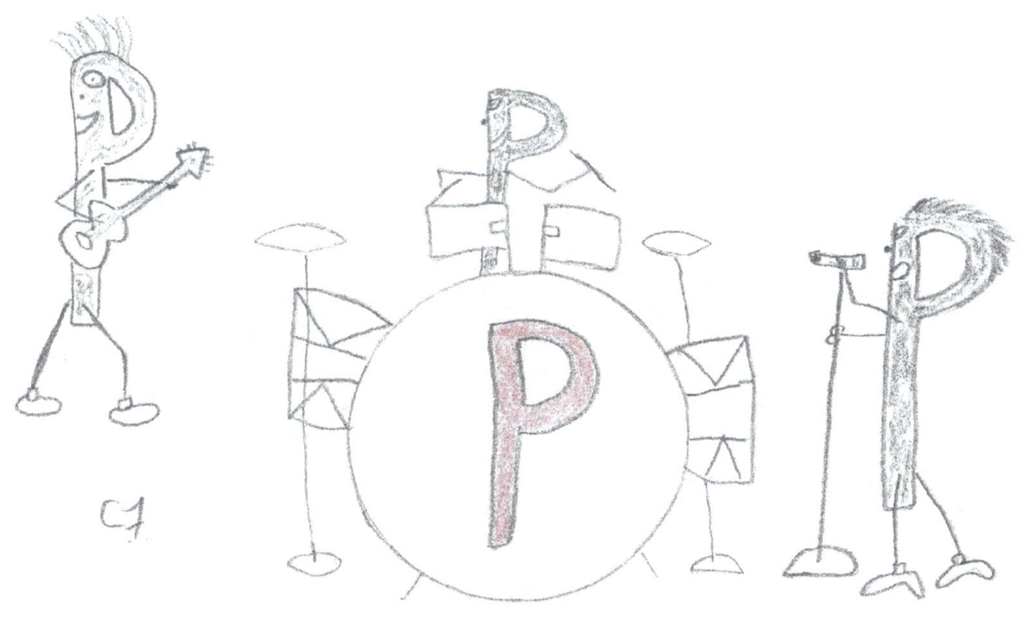

**Go to all your favorite rock concerts,
you already are ahead when moving
to the music!**

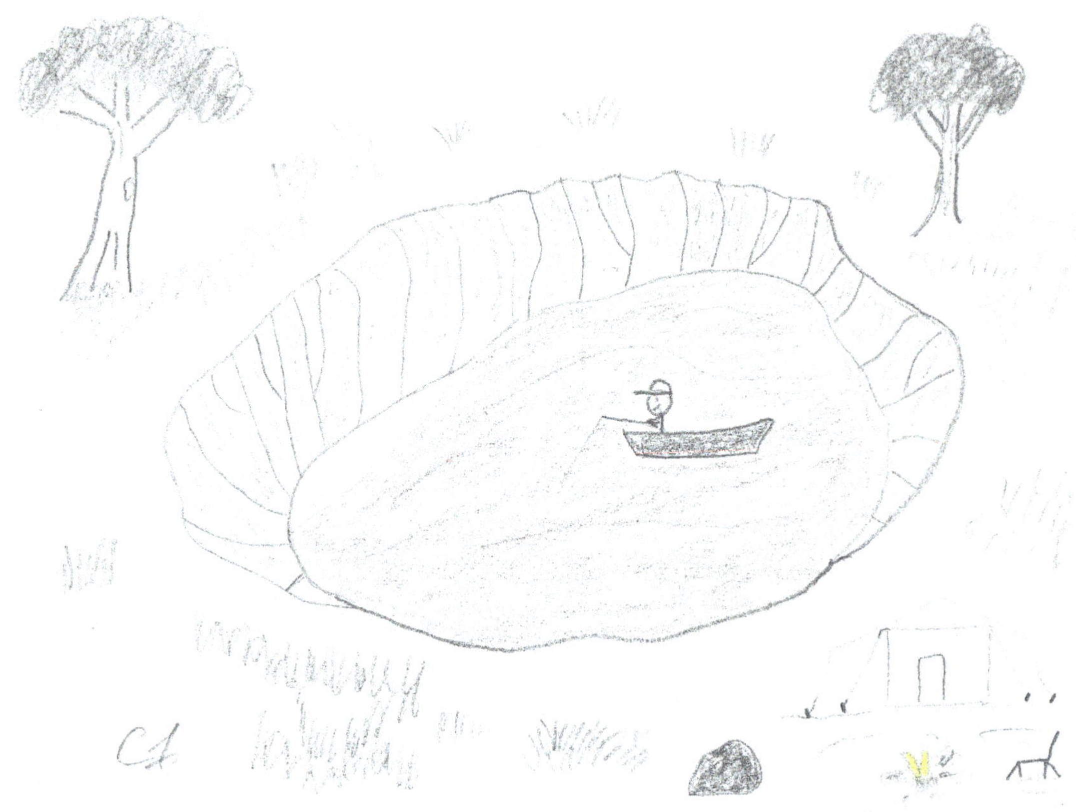

Go Fishing!

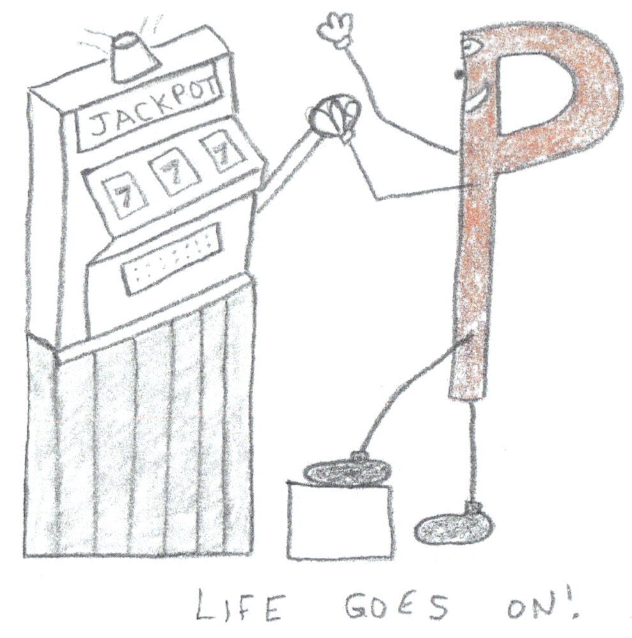

Go win some money!

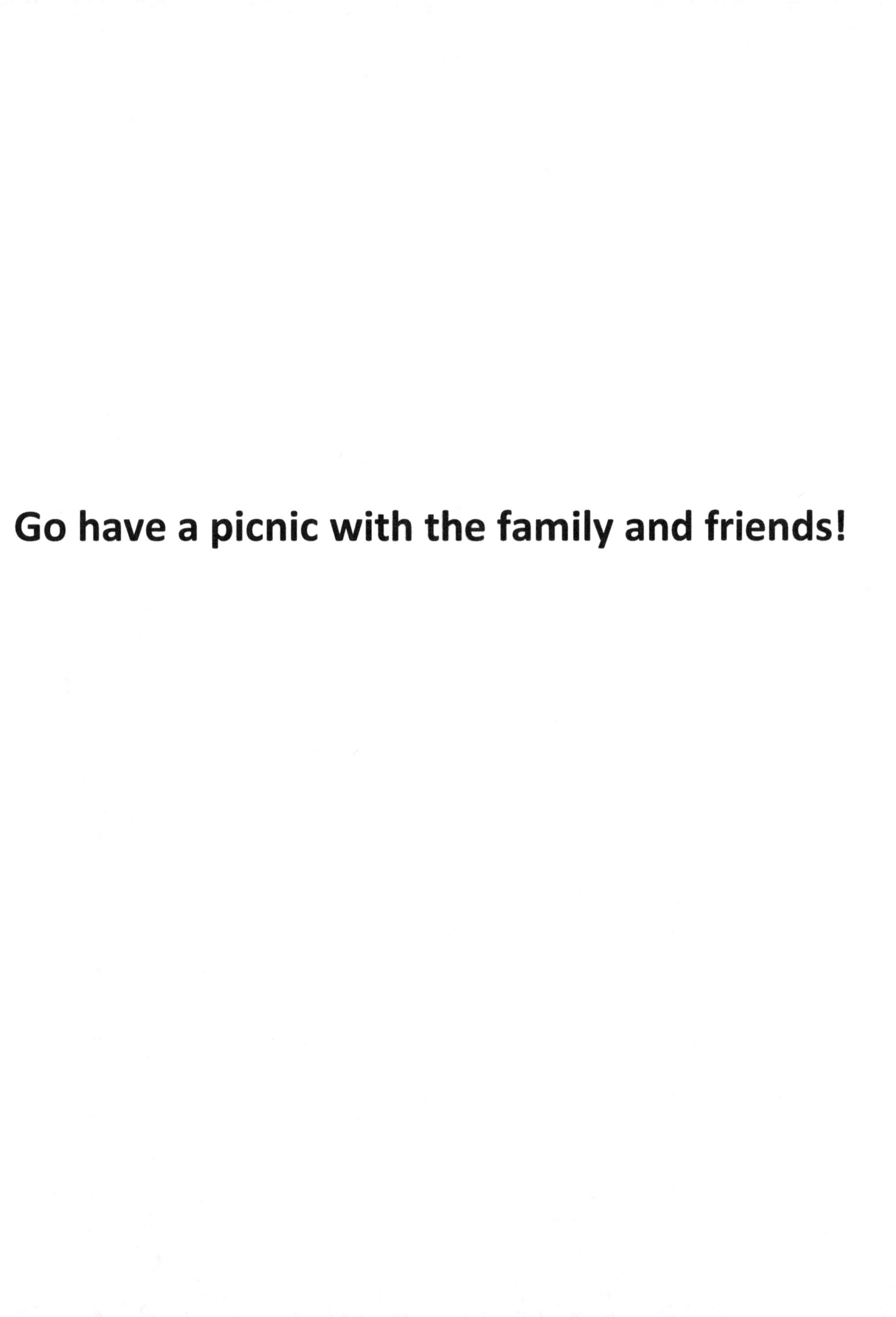
Go have a picnic with the family and friends!

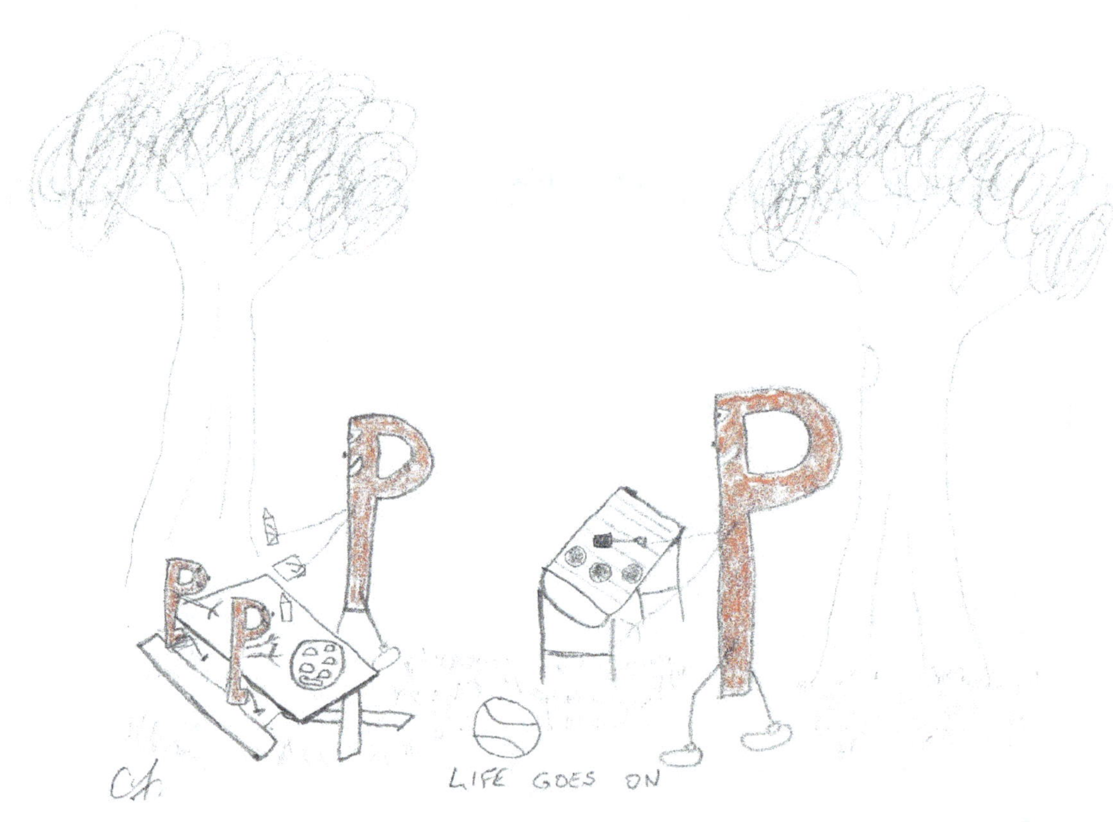

LIFE GOES ON

Life still goes on here in "Shaky Town",
we just "shake" things up some.

Keep on Truckin'!

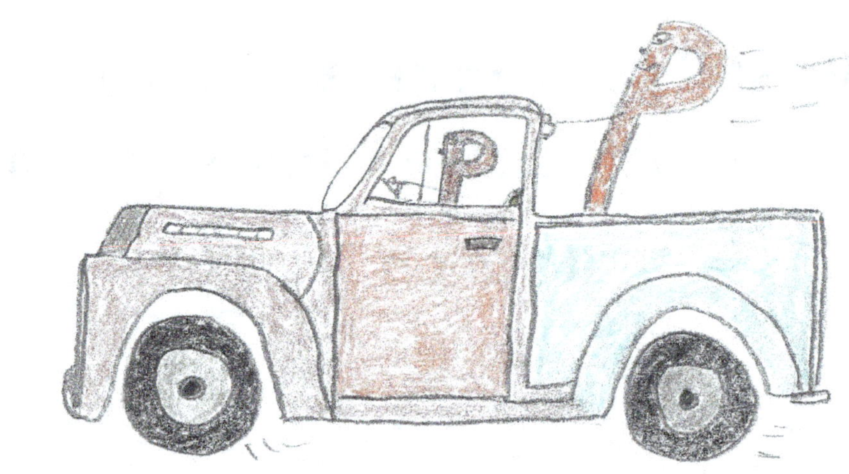

KEEP ON TRUCKIN'

Here are some more pictures I have drawn
for you to enjoy.

PARKINSON'S
GROW'S
ON YOU

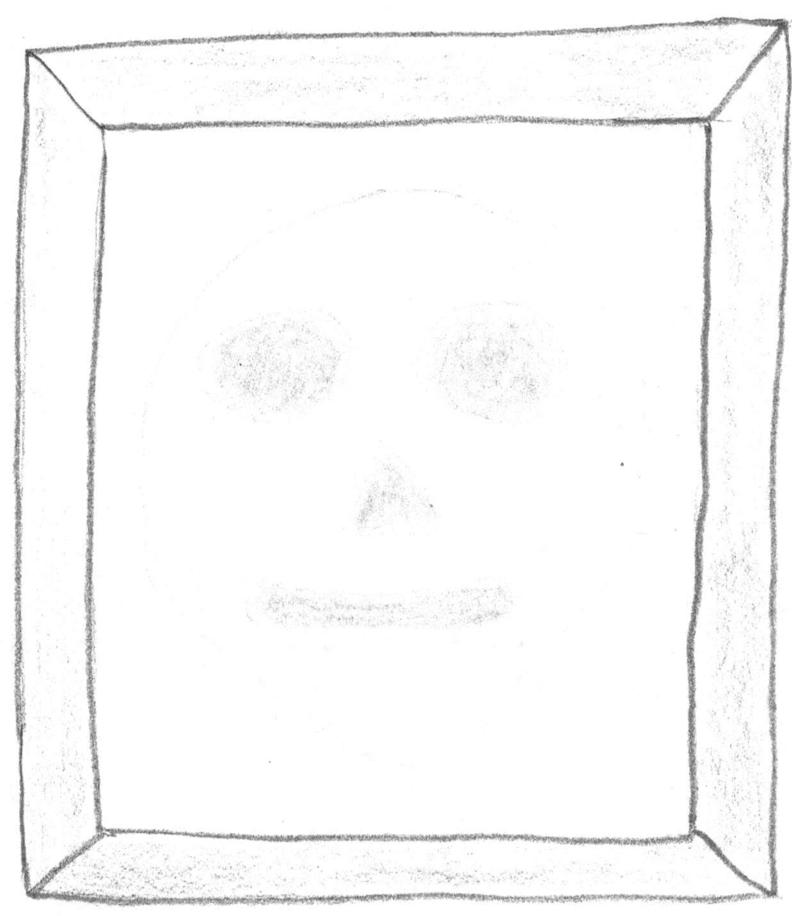

C4 REFLECTION

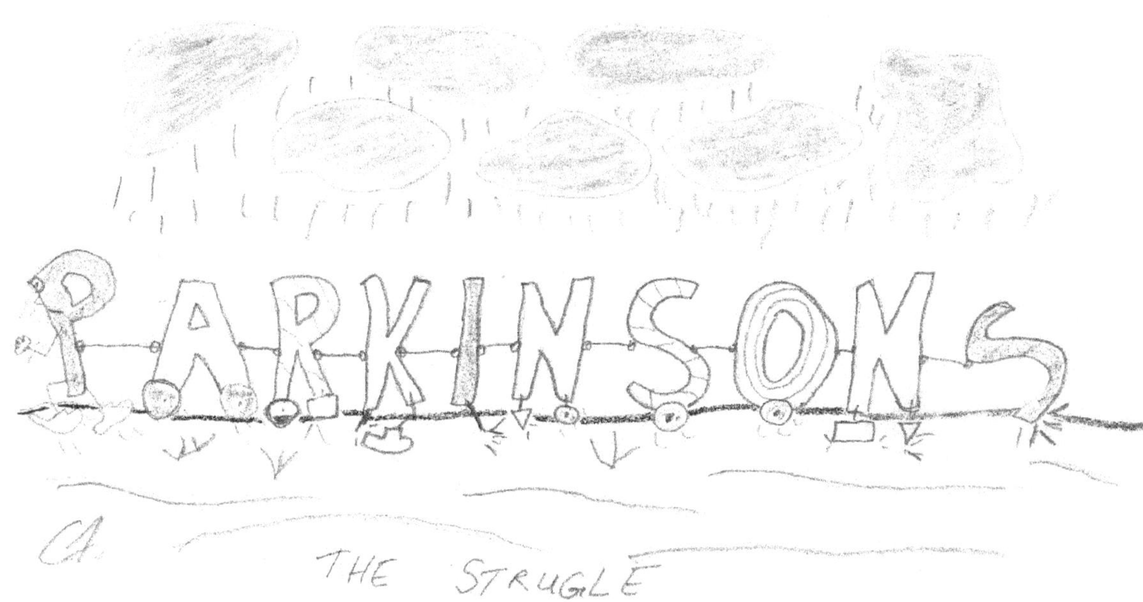

PARKINSONS
THE STRUGLE

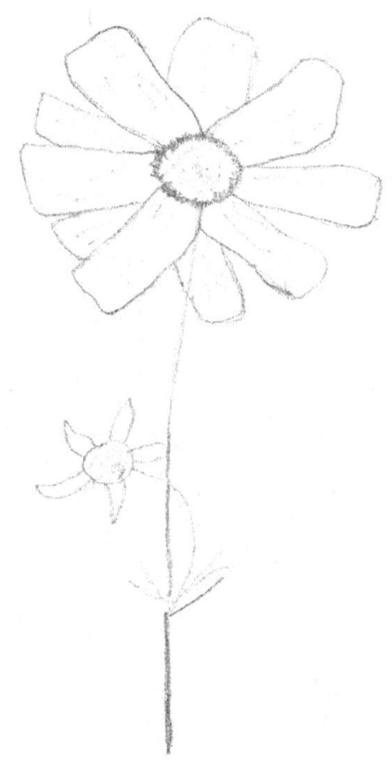

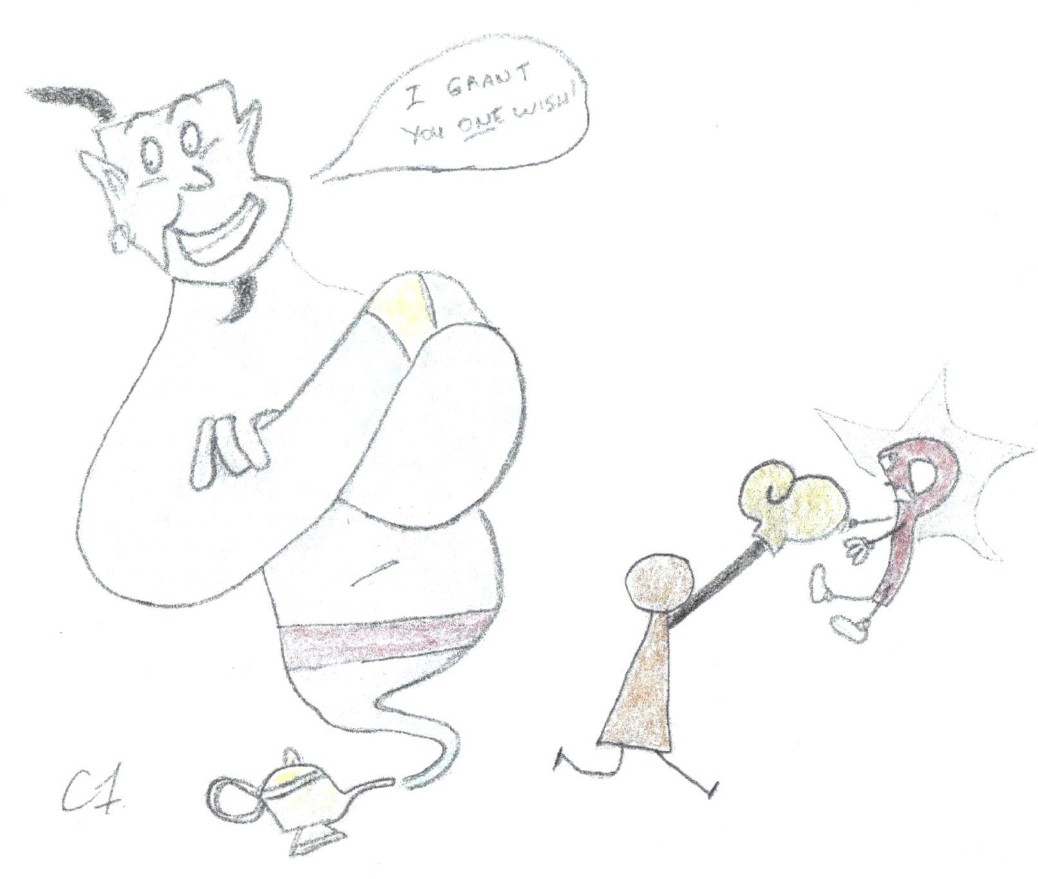

I GRANT YOU ONE WISH!

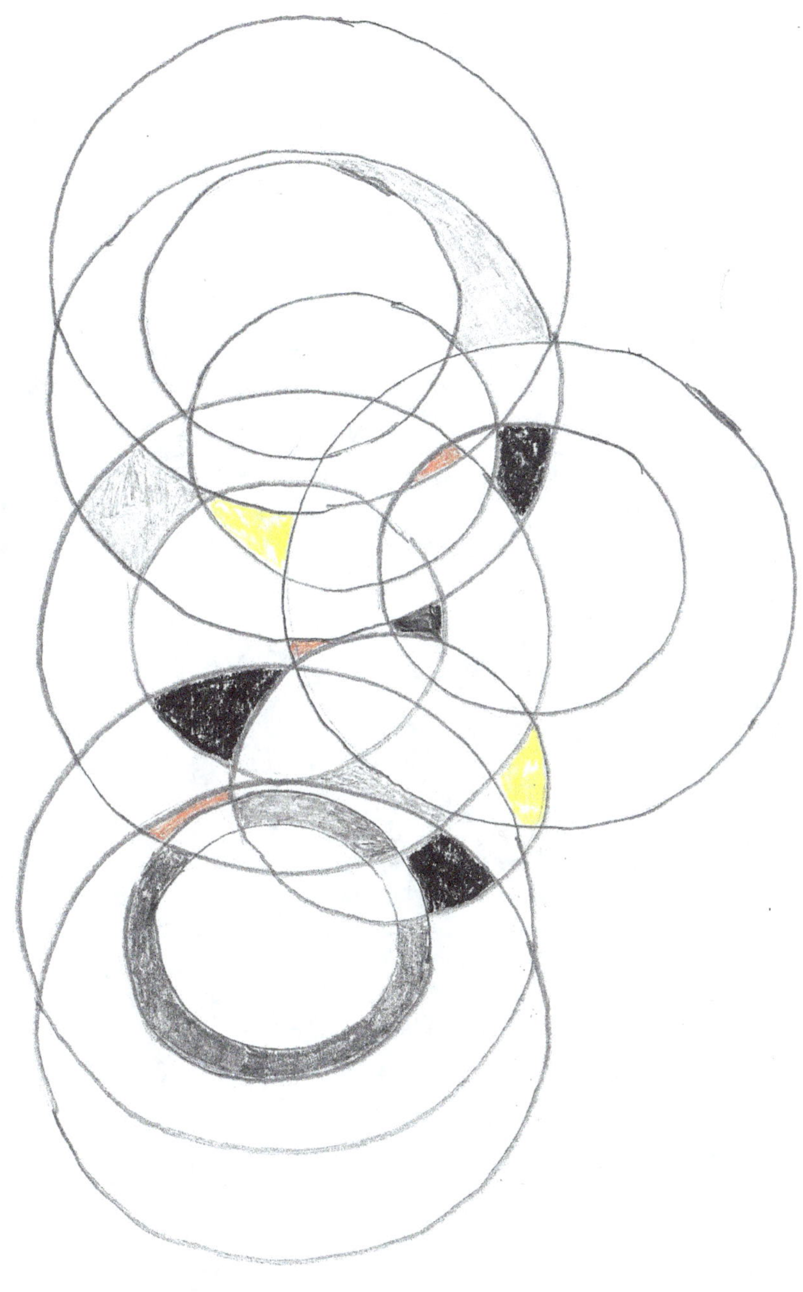

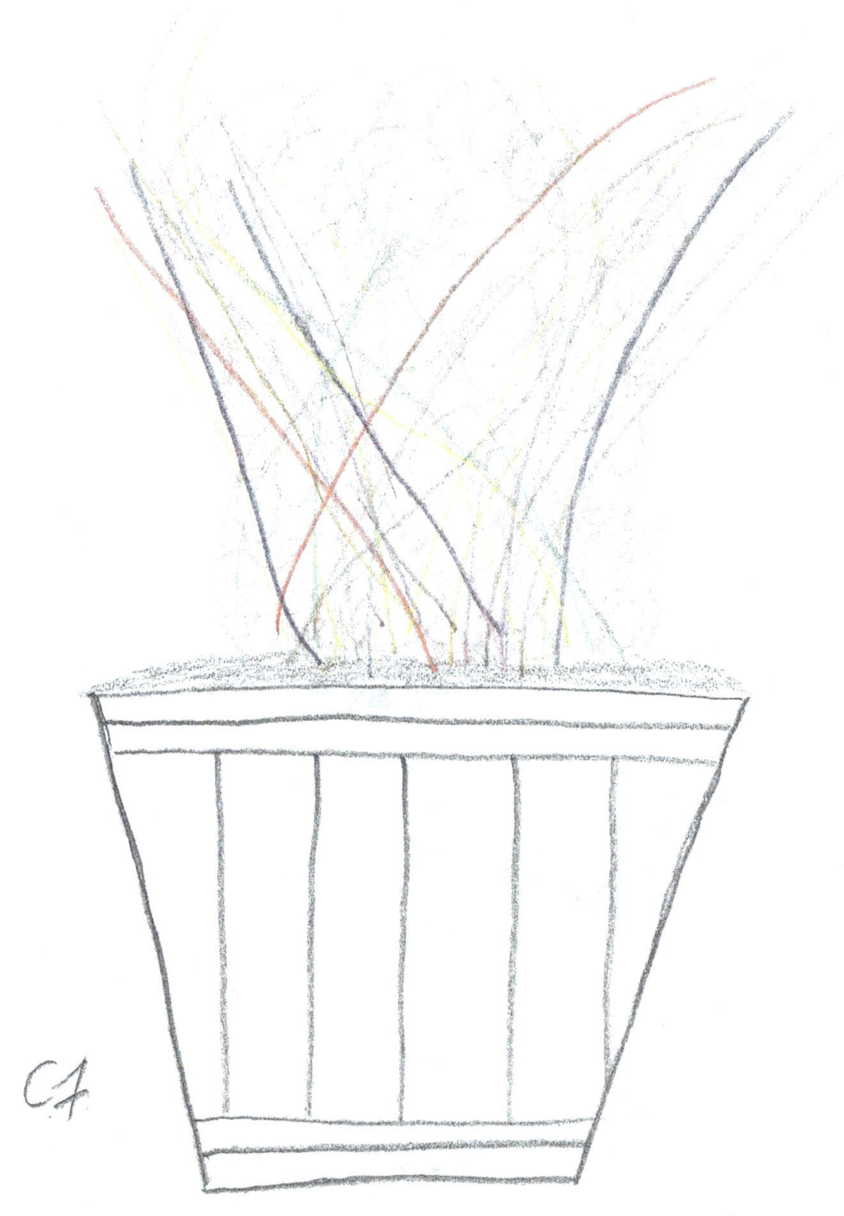

C7

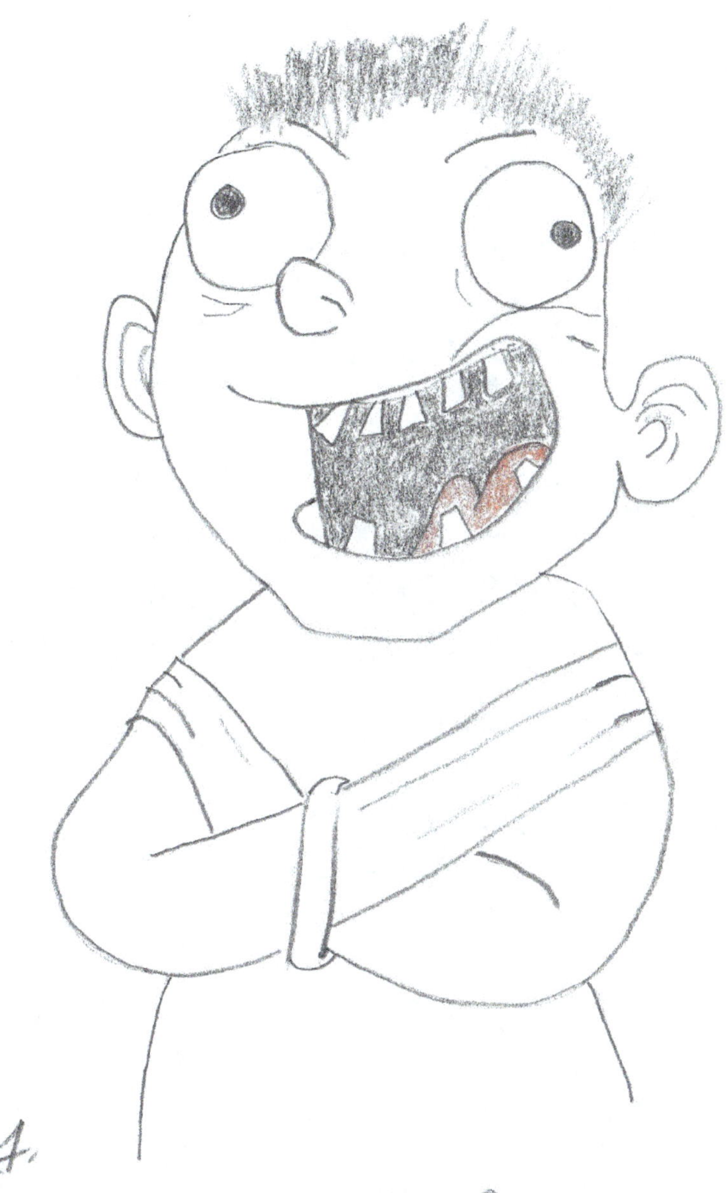

ALL TIED UP

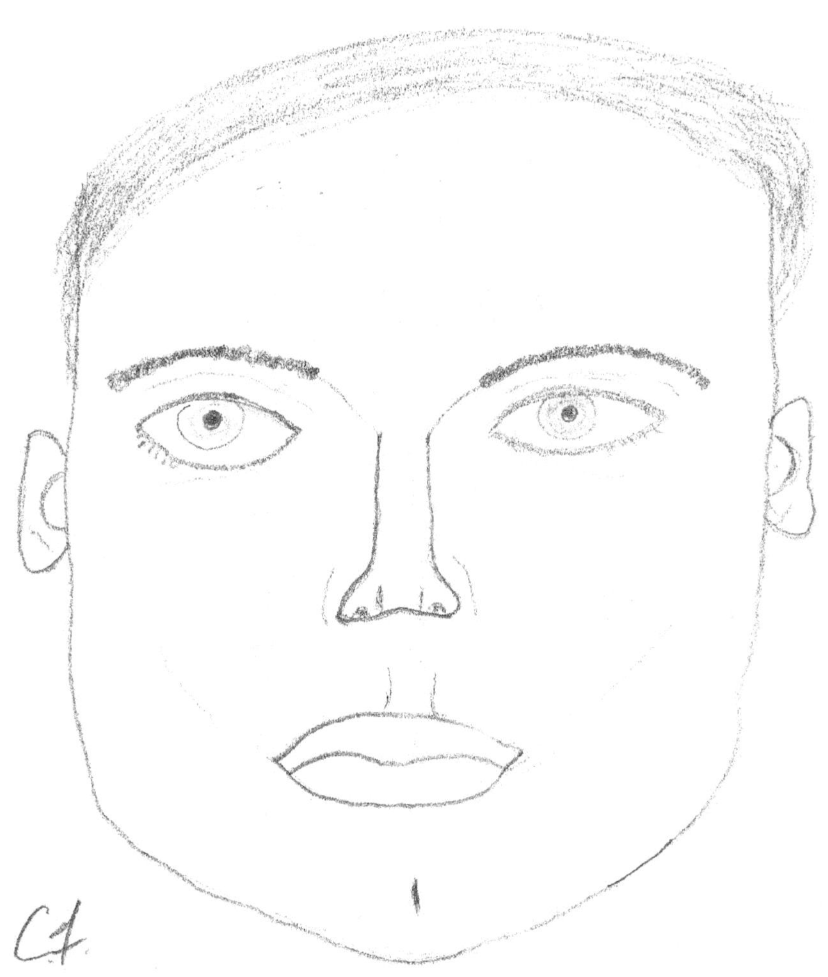

C4.

THE MARK IS MADE

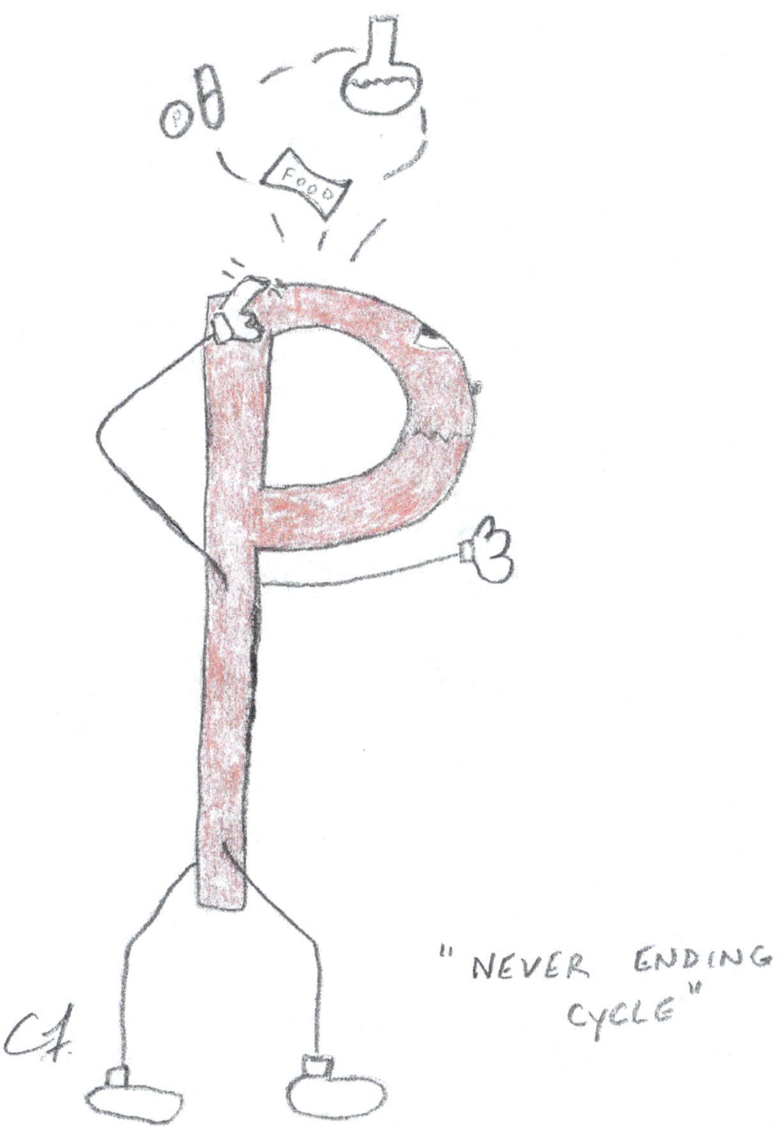

"NEVER ENDING CYCLE"

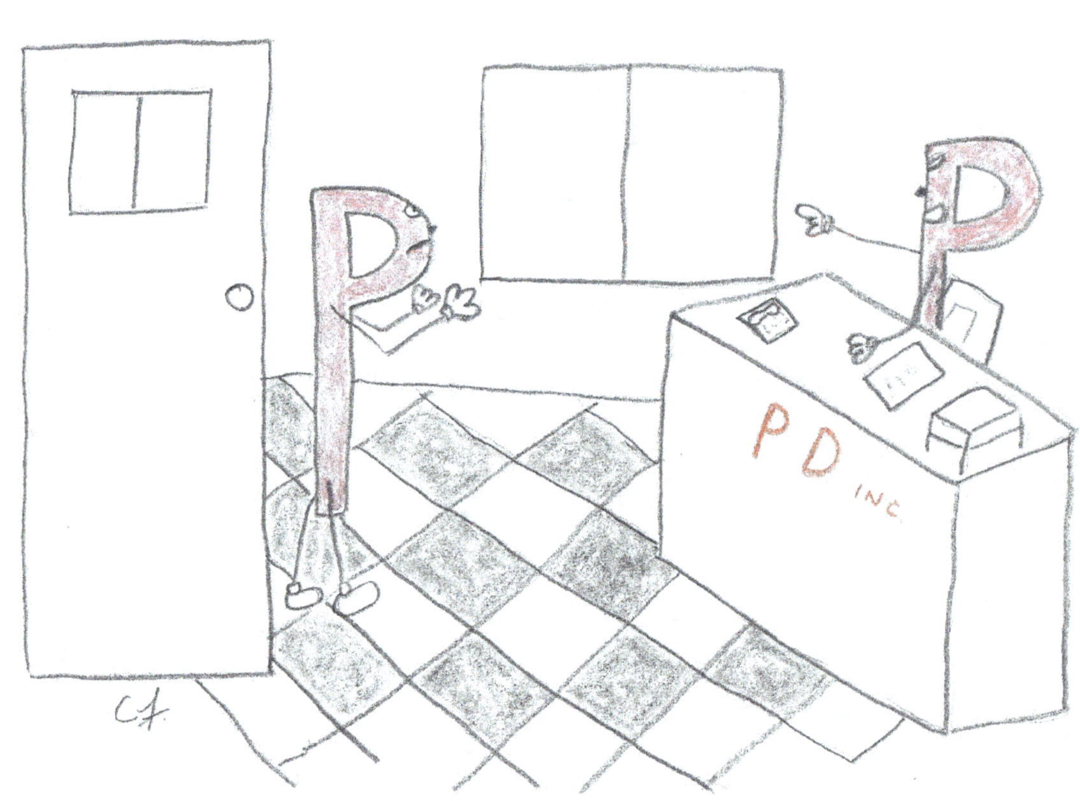

P D INC.

WHAT'S SHAKIN'?

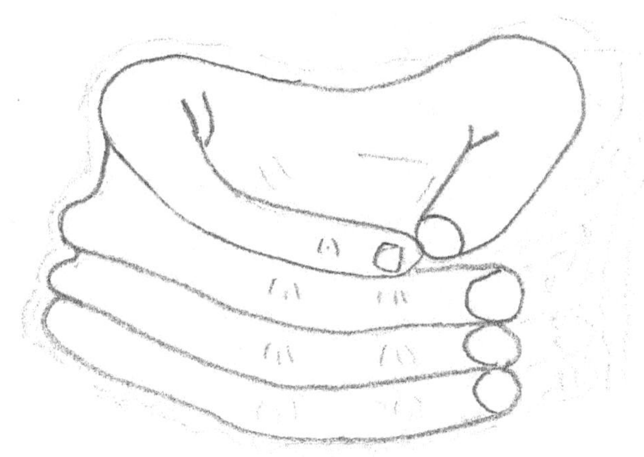

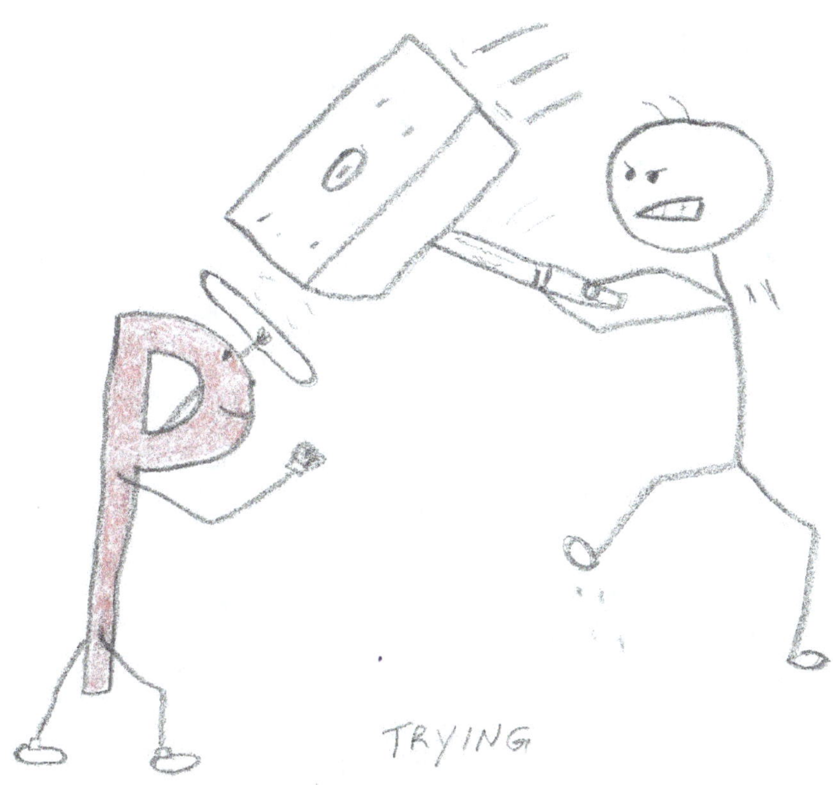

TRYING
C.A.

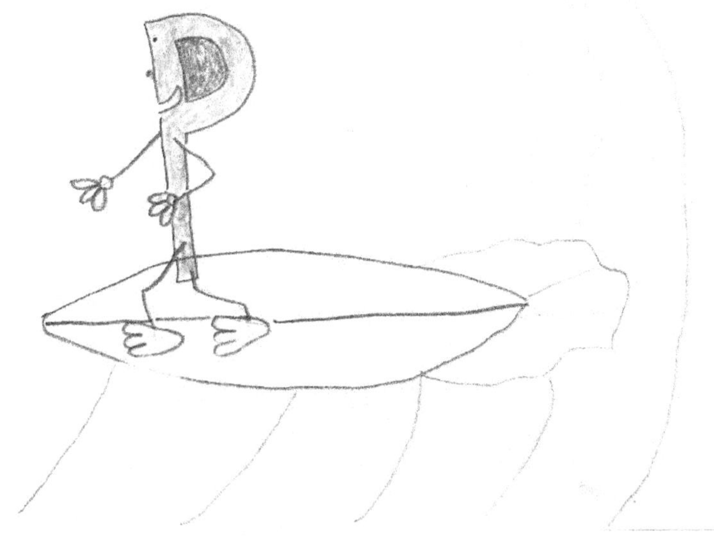

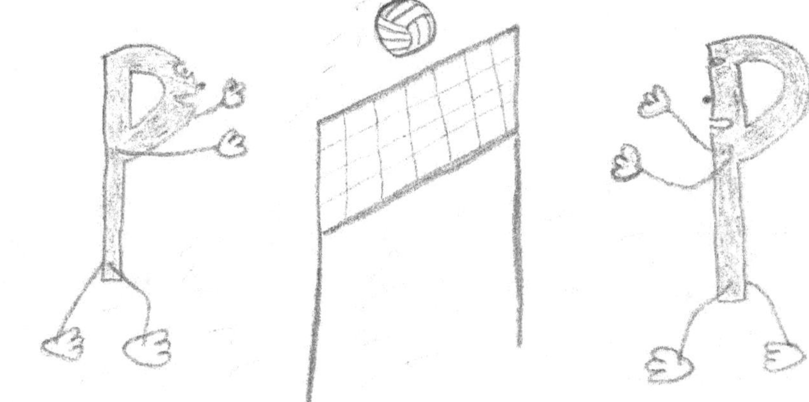

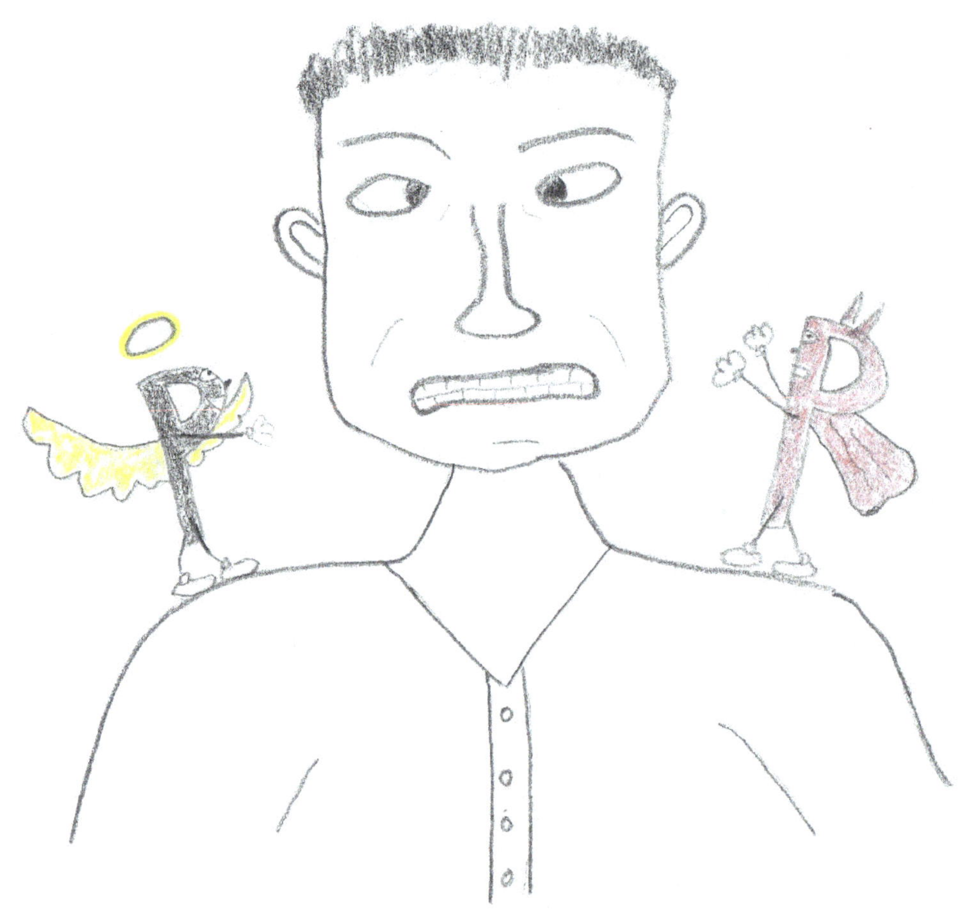

NO MATTER WHAT!

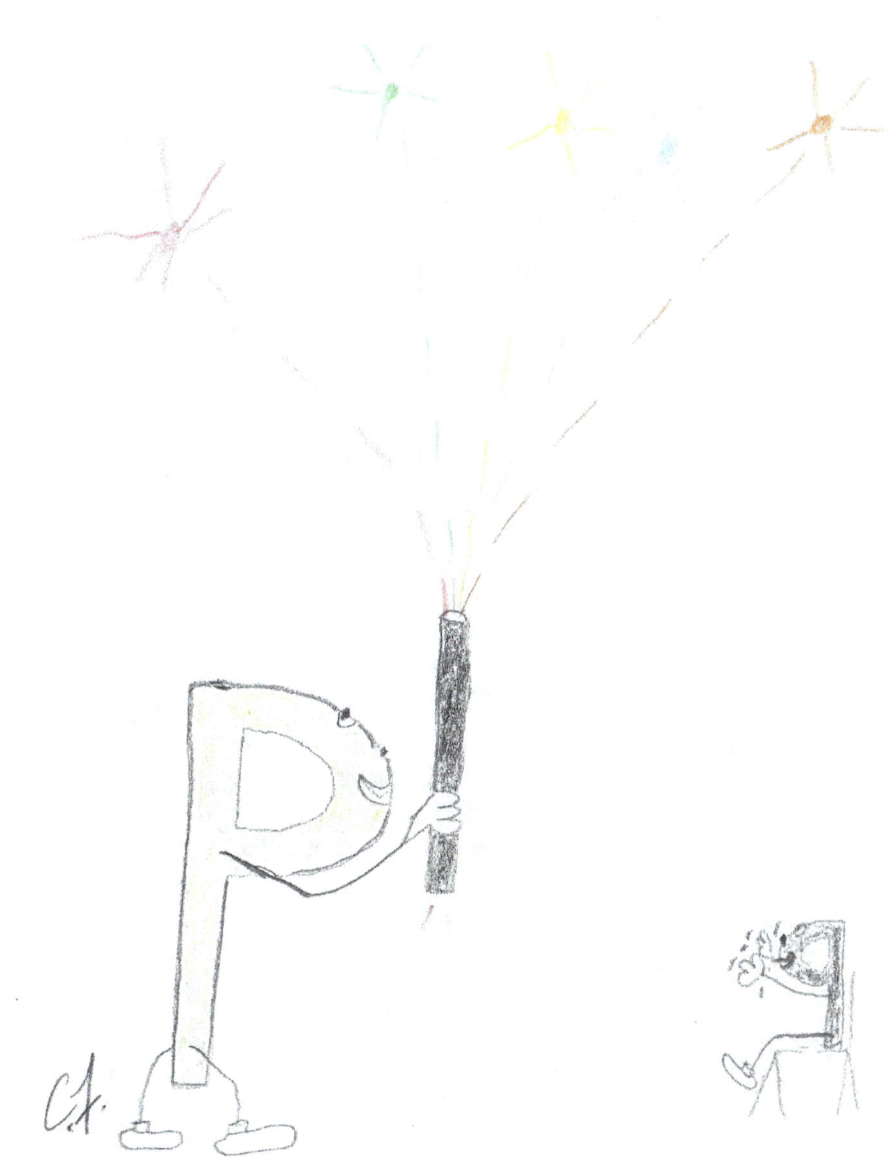

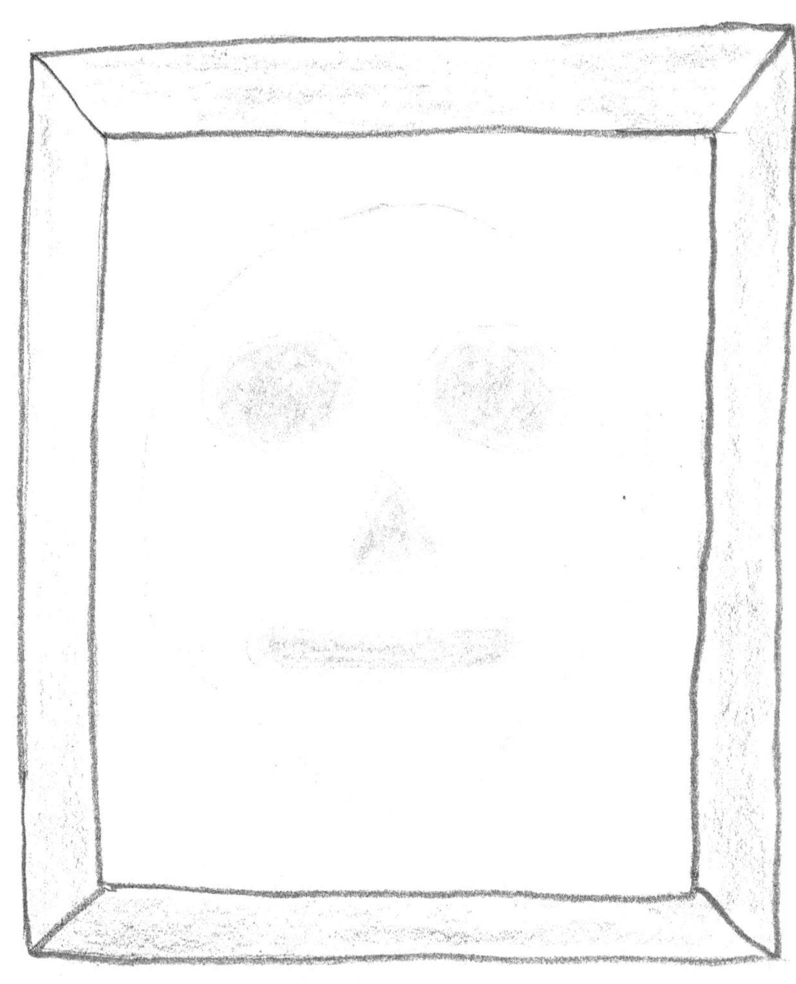

Ct.
REFLECTION

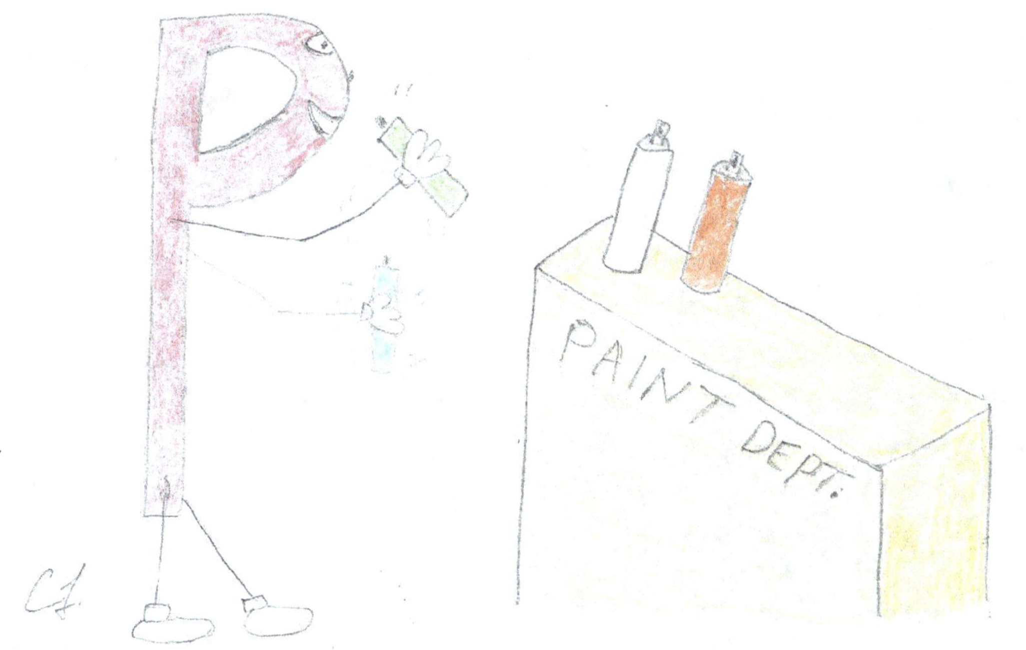
PAINT DEPT.

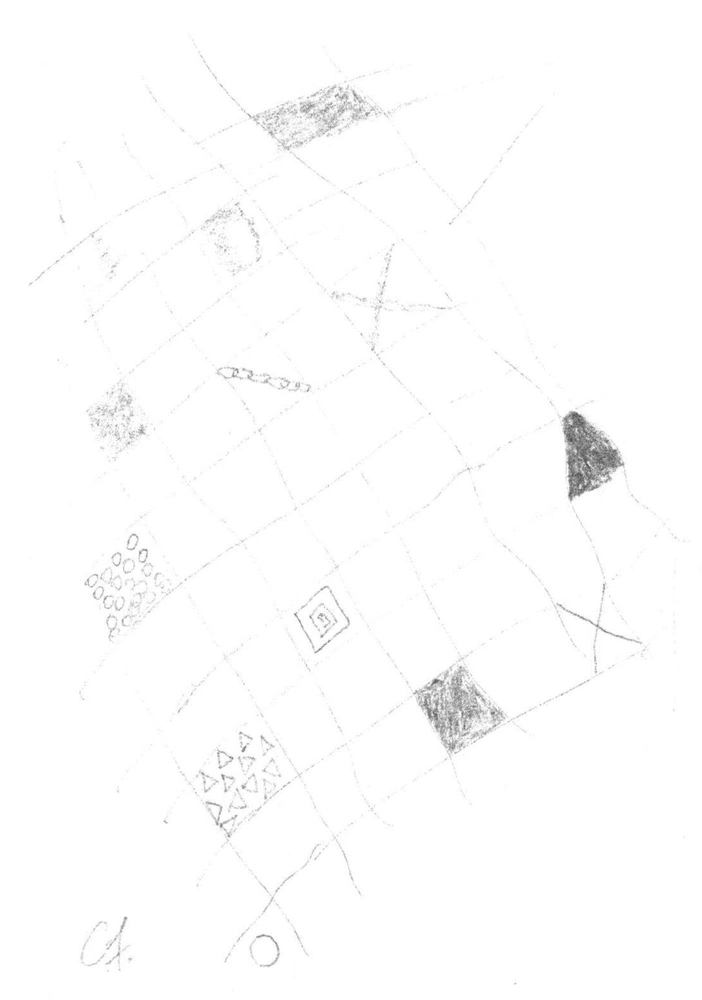

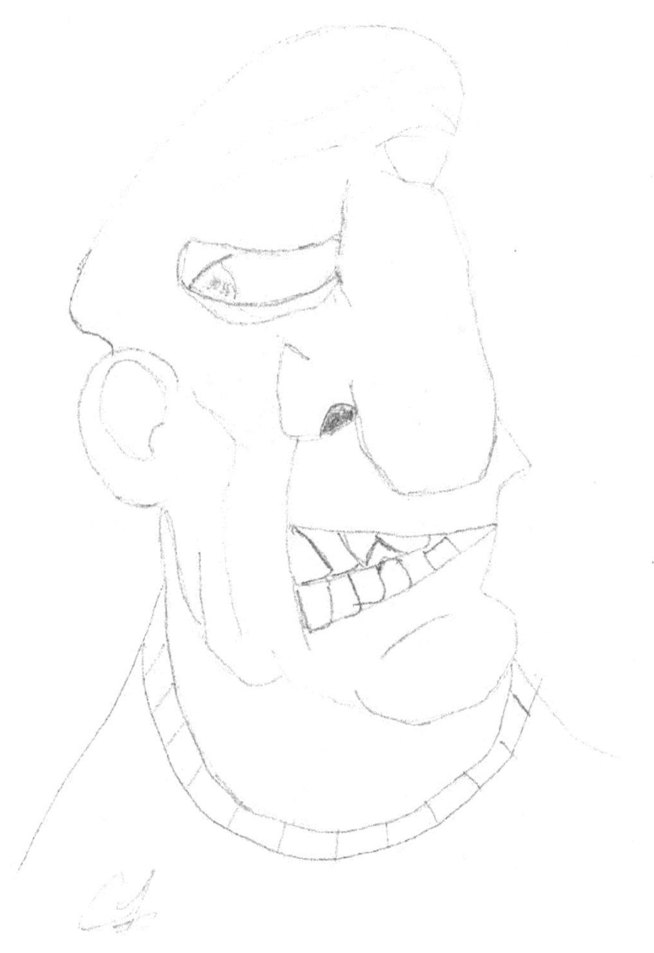

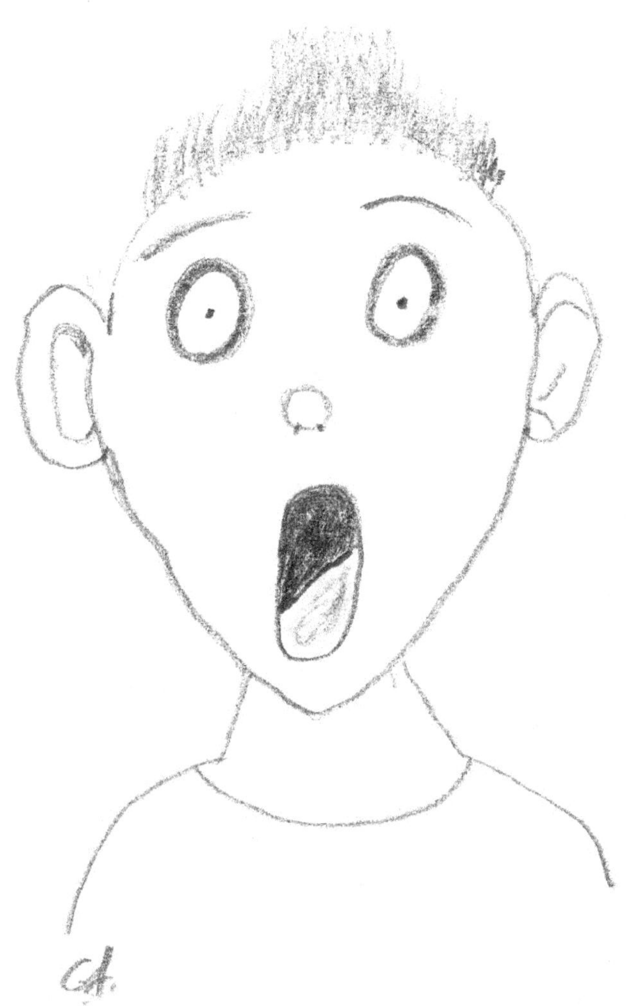

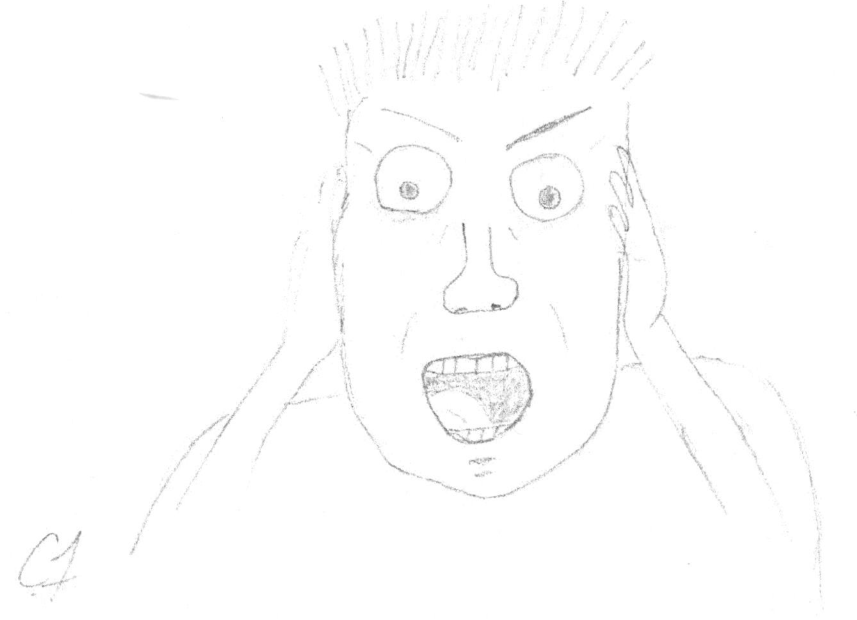

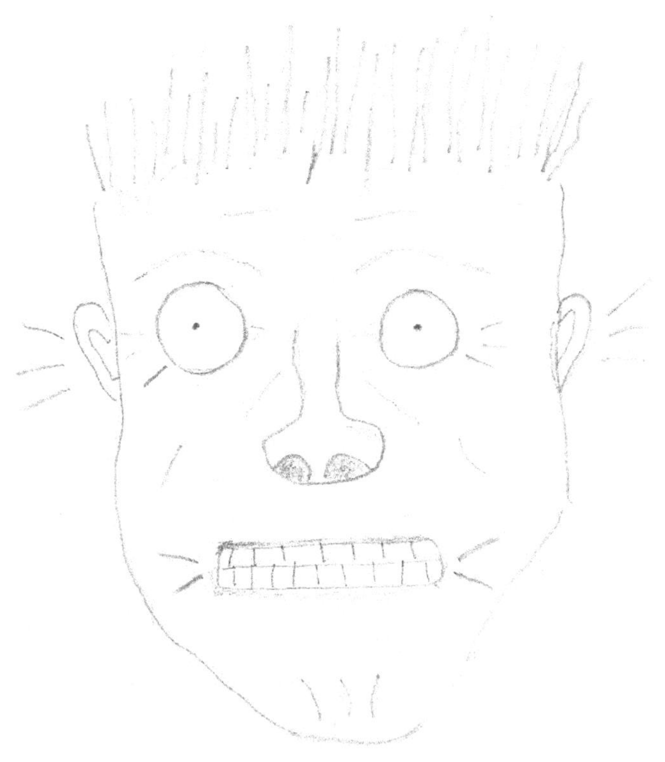

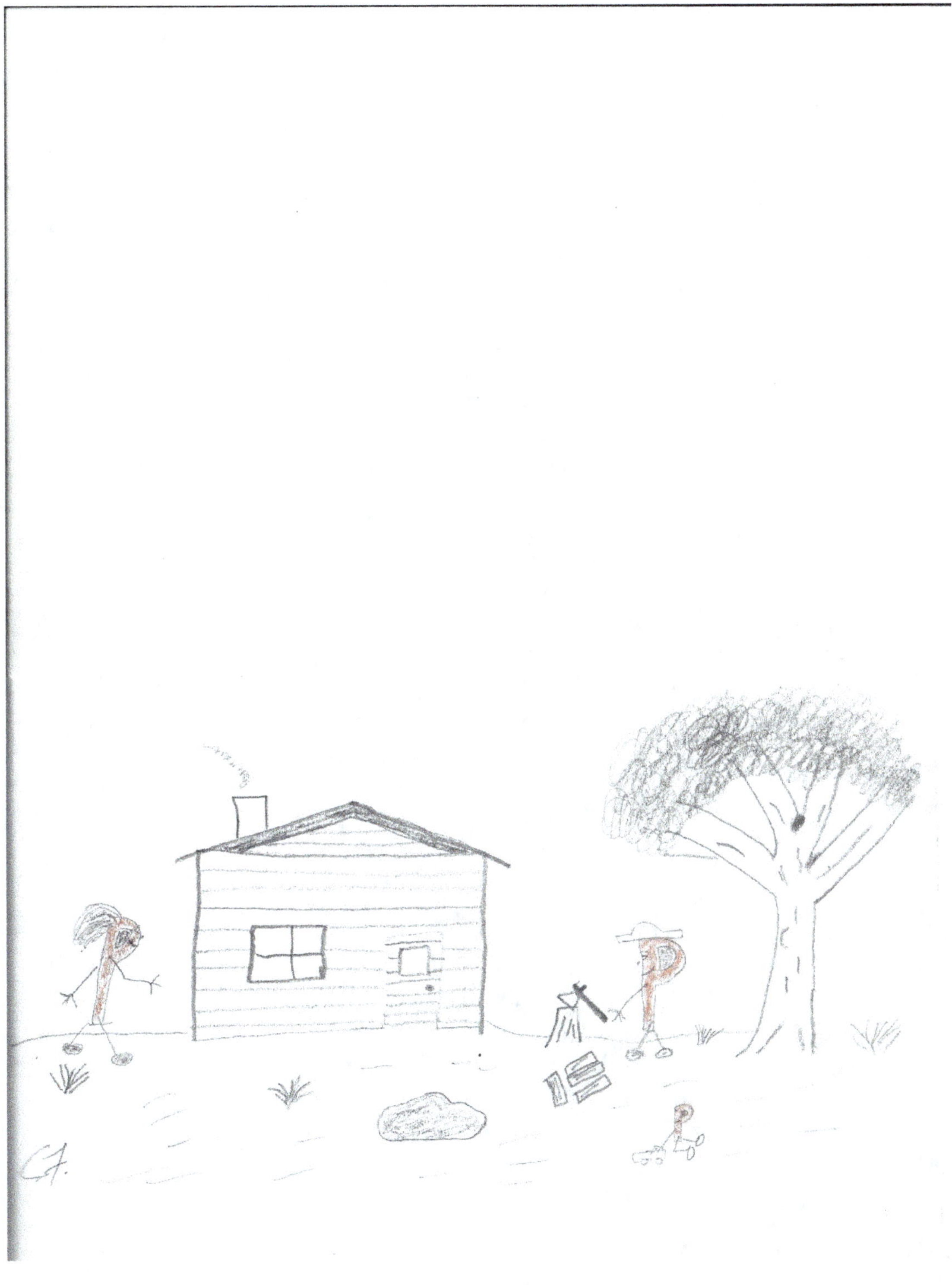

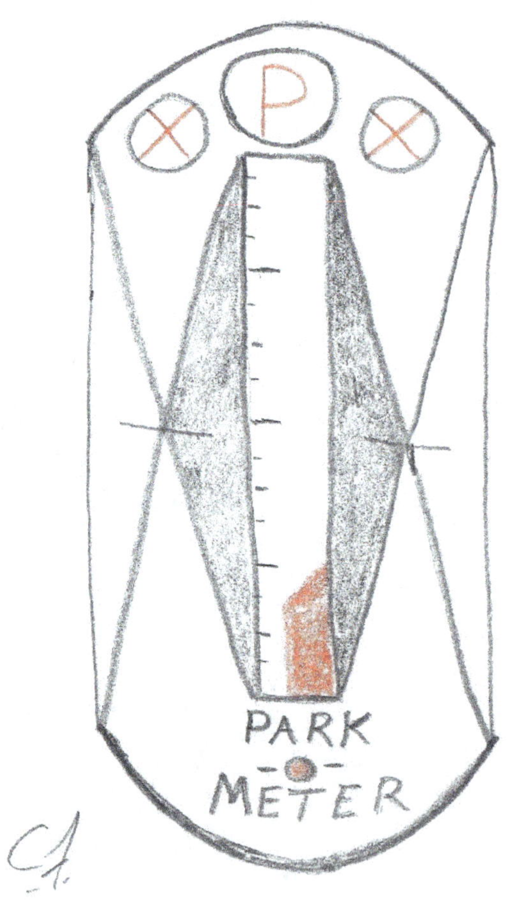

P
X
X
PARK
METER

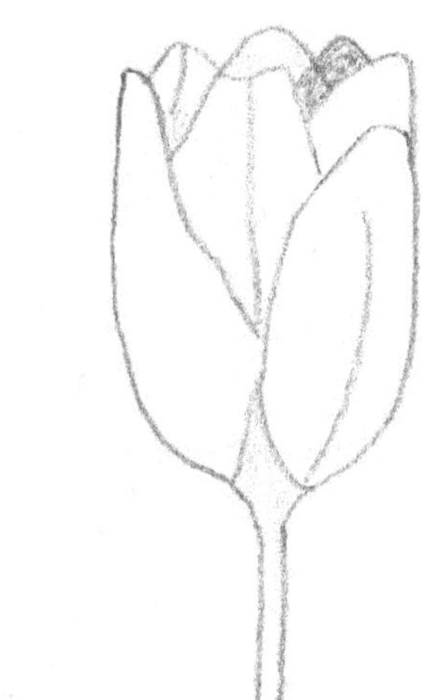
C4

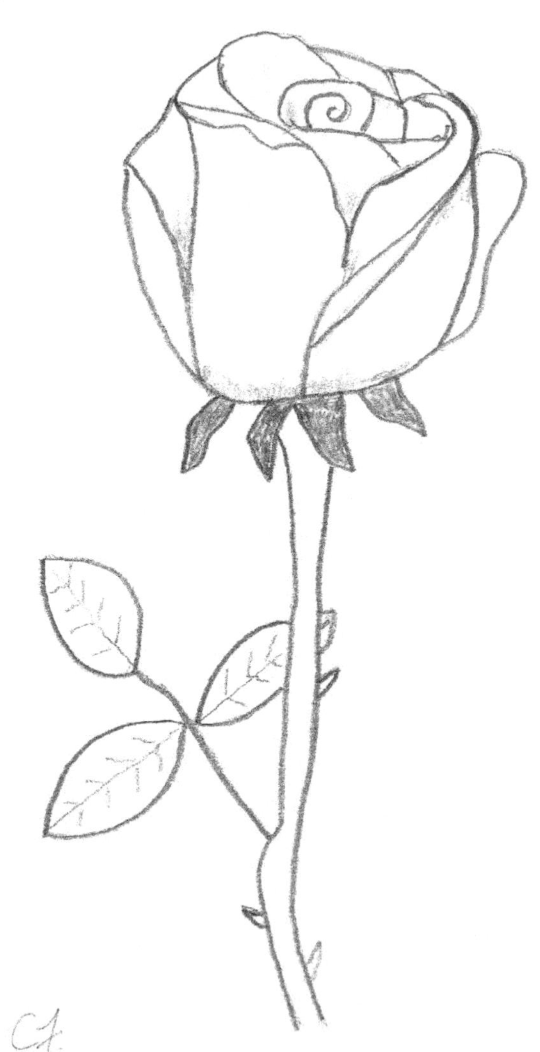

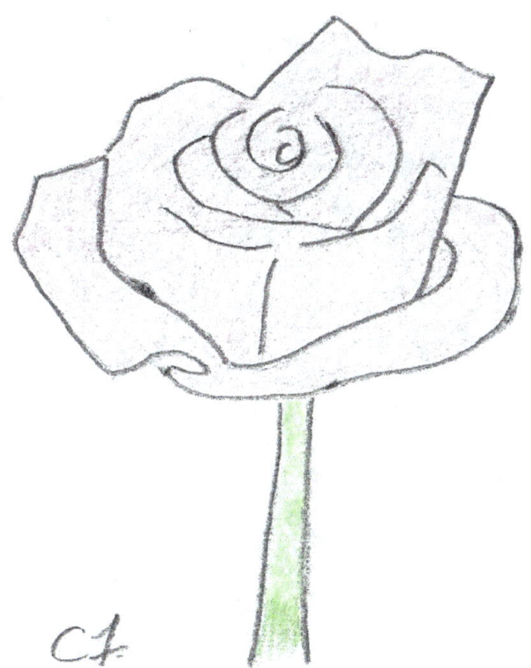

C1.

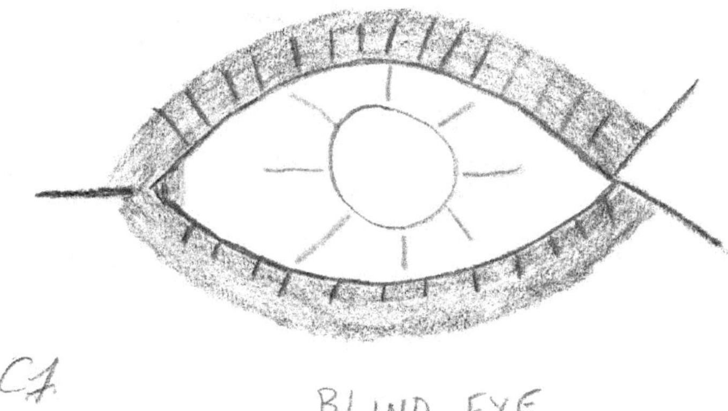

C1.
BLIND EYE

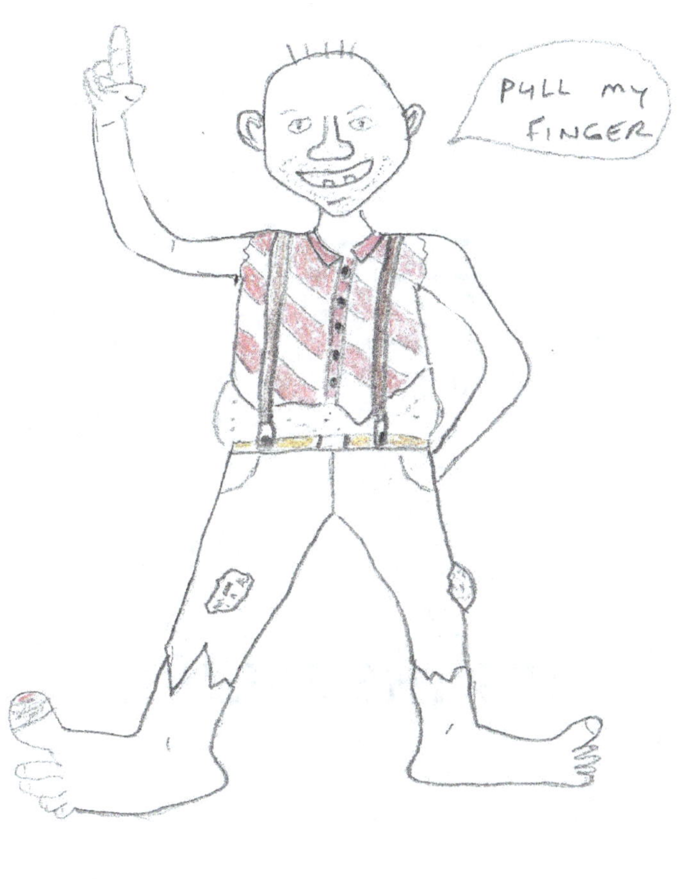

PULL MY FINGER

Thank you for looking at my book and
my drawings.

Hopefully we will be the last generation
to have to deal with this disease!

God Bless!

NOT THE END!!!!!

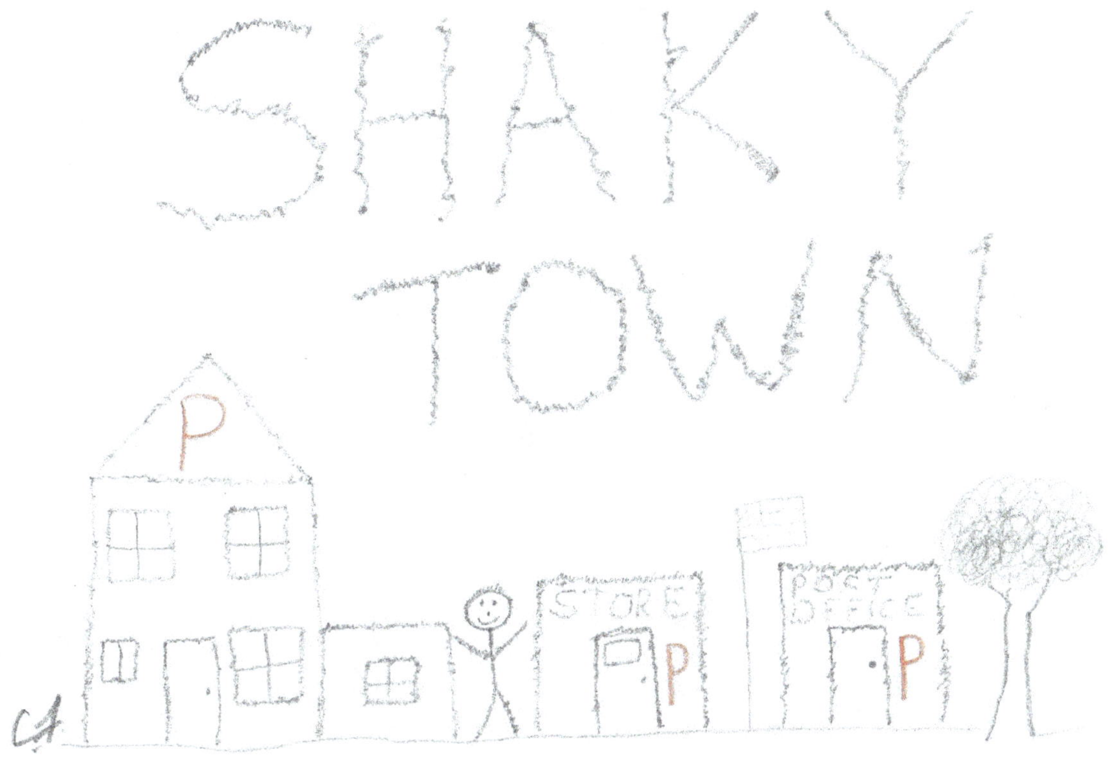

"I have to laugh at Parkinson's because
I refuse to let it make me cry"!